The O[...] [...]

From the Office to the OR

A Guide for the Advanced Care Practitioner

Kenneth A. Egol, MD
Professor and Vice Chair
Department of Orthopaedic Surgery
Hospital for Joint Diseases
NYU Langone Medical Center
New York, New York

Stephanie C. Bazylewicz, PA-C
Physician Assistant
Department of General and Bariatric Surgery
Atlanticare Regional Medical Center
Atlantic City, New Jersey

. Wolters Kluwer

Philadelphia · Baltimore · New York · London
Buenos Aires · Hong Kong · Sydney · Tokyo

Acquisitions Editor: Brian Brown
Editorial Coordinator: Dave Murphy
Marketing Manager: Dan Dressler
Production Project Manager: David Saltzberg
Design Coordinator: Stephen Druding
Manufacturing Coordinator: Beth Welsh
Prepress Vendor: S4Carlisle Publishing Services

9 8 7 6 5 4 3 2 1

Printed in China

Library of Congress Cataloging-in-Publication Data

ISBN-13: 978-1-4963-4457-1
ISBN-10: 1-4963-4457-X

Cataloging in Publication data available on request from publisher.

CCS1017

This book is dedicated to my family, Lori, Alex, Jonathan, and Gabby, for their unending support and to all those who dedicate themselves to be better healthcare providers.

—Kenneth A. Egol

To my husband and parents—thank you for your love, encouragement, and unwavering faith in me. And to all who find themselves treating musculoskeletal conditions they need to learn more about . . . reference your pocket manual and remember, it's going tibia okay.

—Stephanie C. Bazylewicz

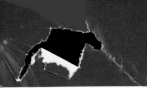

CONTRIBUTORS

Stephanie C. Bazylewicz, PA-C
Physician Assistant
Department of General and
    Bariatric Surgery
Atlanticare Regional Medical
    Center
Atlantic City, New Jersey

Rebekah Belayneh, BA
Medical Student
Howard University School
    of Medicine
Washington, District of Columbia

Kenneth A. Egol, MD
Professor and Vice Chair
Department of Orthopaedic
    Surgery
Hospital for Joint Diseases
NYU Langone Medical Center
New York, New York

David Kugelman, BS
Medical Student
The Commonwealth Medical
    College
Scranton, Pennsylvania

Ariana Lott, BA
Medical Student
University of Pennsylvania School
    of Medicine
Philadelphia, Pennsylvania

Gabrielle C. McIntyre, PA-C
Physician Assistant
Rothman Institute
Galloway, New Jersey

Abdullah Qatu, BSE
Medical Student
New York University School of
    Medicine
New York, New York

Monica Racanelli, MPAS, PA-C
Physician Assistant
Department of Orthopedic
    Surgery
Jamaica Hospital Medical Center
Jamaica, New York

Avraham Schulgasser, PA-C
Physician Assistant
Hospital for Joint Diseases
Department of Orthopaedic
    Surgery
NYU Langone Medical Center
New York, New York

Orthopaedic surgery is the discipline of medicine dedicated to the diagnosis and treatment of conditions affecting the musculoskeletal system inclusive of nerves, tendons, and ligaments. Orthopaedic surgeons and the orthopaedic team use both surgical and nonsurgical means to treat congenital and noncongenital musculoskeletal conditions, including degenerative conditions, musculoskeletal trauma, conditions of the spine, infections, tumors, and sports-related injuries.

The origins of the discipline of orthopaedics date back to the 1700s when Dr Nicolas Andry used the Greek words for "straight" and "child" to form the word "orthopaedic." The discipline expanded to take care of both the pediatric and the adult patient, but the name remained the same. Like many other surgical disciplines, orthopaedics has evolved significantly over the years with much of its evolution taking place around wartime efforts to save life and limb. The battlefield has proven to be a contemporaneous forum for the advancement of orthopaedic treatment measures. Beyond the battlefield, research in orthopaedic care has refined the earliest techniques developed to save life and limb in addition to advancing the field through the study of the role of biomechanics and biomaterials in patient care. Many historical orthopaedic procedures, open cases that had significant comorbid consequences, have evolved to minimally invasive ones with the advent of new technologies.

Modern orthopaedics relies upon an interprofessional orthopaedic team to ensure the appropriate diagnosis and management and to ensure that appropriate medical, nursing, therapeutic, and psychosocial resources are available to each patient. Members of the interprofessional orthopaedic team include the orthopaedist, physician assistants (PAs), nurses, physical therapists (PTs), occupational therapists (OTs), orthopaedic techs, case managers, social workers, dietitians, and others. Each member of the interprofessional orthopaedic team collaborates to play a vital role in achieving the ultimate goal of all orthopaedic patients, which is to restore each patient to maximum functional capacity and quality of life. This is achieved through a holistic approach to patient care with the use of cognitive and technical orthopaedic knowledge, in addition to the use of pharmacotherapeutics, nutritional, and psychosocial services.

The authors of this reference manual are members of the Department of Orthopaedic Surgery at NYU Langone Medical Center, a department affiliated with the care of orthopaedic patients at the Hospital for Joint Diseases. Collectively, these institutions are renowned for excellence in orthopaedic care, research, innovation, and medical education. This manual serves as a reference for members of the orthopaedic team to better understand the multifactorial aspects of caring for the orthopaedic patient. The information within, combined with the collaboration and cooperation of providers and patients, will assist the orthopaedic team in achieving their ultimate goal of restoring each patient to maximum functional capacity and quality of life.

Maureen C. Regan, MBA, PA-C, DFAAPA, FACHE
Administrative Director, Surgical Specialties
NYU Winthrop Hospital
Past President and President-Elect
New York State Society of Physician Assistants
Delegate, American Academy of Physician Assistants

PREFACE

Advanced practice provers of musculoskeletal care include physician assistants (PAs) and nurse practitioners (NPs) who provide high-quality, cost-effective health care. These nonphysician orthopaedic providers work in concert with orthopaedic surgeons' and physiatrists as important members of the orthopaedic care team to help those with musculoskeletal complaints.

The idea for this book arose from our experience with advanced practice provers at our orthopaedic specialty hospital. During the course of teaching these nonphysician health care providers the basics of many of the orthopaedic office and operating room procedures, it became clear to us that no concise text was available to aid in the process. With the demand for musculoskeletal care continuing to increase, the nonphysician orthopaedic provider will be called upon to play an ever-expanding role in the delivery of orthopaedic care. While the basic type of knowledge is available to practitioners in large expansive texts and online resources, we felt that a pocket manual with coverage of a wide variety of musculoskeletal conditions, procedures, and paperwork references required in today's health care would be a useful reference for treating orthopaedic patients in a variety of settings.

This manual has been prepared in a manner that will aid any musculoskeletal practitioner in any practice setting, as well as any nonphysician health care provider who is charged with attending to patients presenting to the emergency department with an acute traumatic musculoskeletal complaint in need of intervention. Despite the ever-increasing expanse of knowledge within the medical field, this book focuses on those aspects of musculoskeletal care that an Advanced practice provider (APP) will commonly treat. This first-edition, pocket-sized guide contains the necessary information to be used as a reference in the office and the operating room. We hope that the users of this book find it useful in their daily care of patients with musculoskeletal complaints.

Kenneth A. Egol, MD
Stephanie C. Bazylewicz, PA-C

ACKNOWLEDGMENTS

We would like to thank Oriana Rivera for her artistic talent.

Kenneth A. Egol, MD
Stephanie C. Bazylewicz, PA-C

CONTENTS

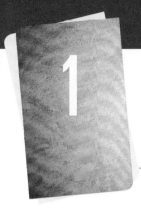

1

THE SPECIALTY OF ORTHOPAEDIC SURGERY

Abdullah Qatu and Kenneth A. Egol

I. THE MUSCULOSKELETAL SYSTEM

The function of the musculoskeletal system is to provide support and stability in a manner that is conducive for movement of the human body and protection of its vital organs. It is the main reservoir of calcium and phosphorus as well as the site for hematopoietic differentiation. This system of mesodermic origin consists predominantly of bone and muscle bound together by various connective tissue elements that include ligaments and tendons.[1]

Bone

There are 206 bones in a normal adult classified in 3 general categories: long bones, short bones, and flat bones. These bones interact via connective tissue elements to form the skeleton, which is further divided into the axial skeleton (skull, rib cage, and vertebral column) and the appendicular skeleton (limbs, shoulder girdle, and pelvic girdle).[1]

Bone development occurs in two ways: endochondral or intramembranous ossification. Endochondral ossification occurs primarily in long and short bones such that chondrocytes form a cartilaginous model and osteoblasts and osteoclasts remodel this to mature lamellar bone.[2] Endochondral ossification of long bones eventually gives rise to three anatomic zones referred to as the epiphysis, metaphysis, and diaphysis (Figure 1-1). Intramembranous ossification occurs primarily in flat bones such that immature bone is formed without a cartilaginous model and is subsequently remodeled into mature, lamellar bone.[1]

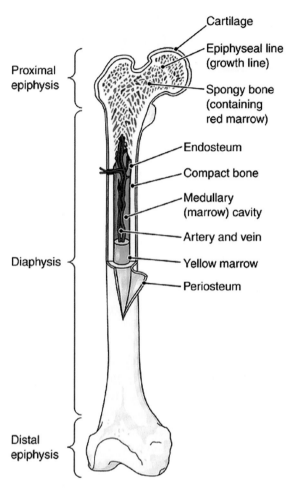

Figure 1-1 Schematic of long bone anatomy. Schematic of long bone delineating physeal zones along with outer and inner anatomy. (From Cohen BJ, Hull KL. *Memmler's Structure and Function of the Human Body*. Philadelphia, PA: Wolters Kluwer Health/Lippincott Williams & Wilkins; 2015.)

The entire bone is covered by periosteum. Beneath the periosteum are three layers of bone, the most superficial of which is cortical. Underneath the cortical bone lies the cancellous bone, which surrounds the medullary cavity (Figure 1-1). The periosteum is an innervated and highly vascularized dense connective tissue. Cortical (compact) bone forms the bone's exterior and comprises up to 80% of the skeleton. Its fundamental functional unit is the osteon or Haversian system. The osteon is a series of concentric layers of mineralized matrix surrounding a central canal (Haversian canal), which provides a tract for vascular and nerve supply. Each concentric layer contains a ring of spaces called lacunae that house the osteocyte cell responsible for maintaining bone homeostasis. Cancellous (trabecular or spongy) bone has a less organized, trabecular structure with a higher surface area to mass ratio than cortical bone and is predominantly found at the end of long bones. It is highly vascularized, less dense, weaker, and more elastic than cortical bone. Normal cortical and cancellous bone is referred to as lamellar bone and is stress oriented in configuration. This composite nature of bone gives rise to its viscoelastic property such that its strain is time dependent when undergoing deformation. Lastly, the innermost medullary cavity is the site of hematopoietic stem cell differentiation.[1]

Bone is a dynamic tissue that consists of a mineralized organic matrix that is highly regulated by its cellular components. Osteoblasts act to synthesize and deposit the organic component of bone matrix called osteoid, which consists predominantly of type 1 collagen. Osteoid is eventually mineralized to hydroxyapatite consisting predominantly of calcium and phosphate. Osteoclasts act to break down bone in a process called bone resorption. Resorption occurs with osteoclasts tightly clinging onto the bone surface and secreting acids to dissolve the mineral matrix along with collagenases and other enzymes to break down the organic components. It is essential to maintain homeostasis between osteoclast and osteoblast activity.

Osteoblasts are key regulators of this balance because they act to modulate osteoclast activity. For example, in response to hypocalcemia, the parathyroid gland will release parathyroid hormone (PTH) to increase serum calcium levels chiefly through bone resorption. PTH receptors, however, are located on osteoblasts, which will subsequently act to differentiate and activate osteoclast precursors for resorption when stimulated. This is mediated by osteoblast surface expression of the extracellular membrane protein RANKL (Receptor Activator of Nuclear factor-Kappa B Ligand). Osteoclast precursor cells contain RANK receptors on their membranes that allow them to differentiate into mature osteoclast cells capable of resorption when bound to RANKL (Figure 1-2). Osteoclast precursor cells contain RANK receptors on their membranes that allow them to differentiate into mature osteoclast cells capable of resorption. Osteoblasts additionally secrete osteoprotegerin, which acts to bind RANKL and prevents its interaction with the RANK receptor and prevents osteoclast differentiation when necessary for homeostatic control. It is, therefore, the ratio of secreted osteoprotegerin to RANKL expression by osteoblasts that dictates the degree of bone resorption. PTH is one of many factors that induce osteoclast activation.[1]

Healthy bone is constantly being remodeled by osteoblast and osteoclast activity. Wolff's law states that this remodeling occurs in response to mechanical stress in order to adapt to these loads. Thus, an increase in mechanical stress will increase bone deposition, whereas the lack of mechanical stress results in bone loss. For

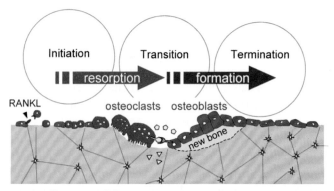

Figure 1-2 Bone remodeling. A schematic example of the process of bone remodeling. Osteoblasts expressing RANKL activate osteoclast resorption while osteoblasts form new bone. (Courtesy of Thorston Kirsch, PhD.)

example, owing to the lack of a gravitational stress, astronauts are prone to bone loss in space.[1]

Skeletal Muscle

Skeletal muscle is one of the three types of muscle found in the body and is responsible for voluntary movement. The skeletal muscle cell, or fiber, is multinucleate and cylindrical in shape with a plasma membrane referred to as the sarcolemma. Each fiber contains a plethora of myofibrils, which are most importantly composed of actin, myosin, and titin. These myofibrils are systematically arranged into thick and thin filaments, which are further organized into a series of repeating sections called the sarcomere across the entire length of the myofibril (Figure 1-3). It is this pattern that gives skeletal

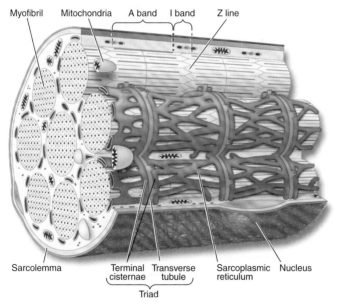

Figure 1-3 Cross section of skeletal muscle sarcomere. Cross section of skeletal muscle demonstrating muscle fibers, myofibrils, and sarcomere organization. (From McArdle WD, Katch FI, Katch VL. *Essentials of Exercise Physiology.* 2nd ed. Baltimore, MD: Lippincott Williams and Wilkins; 2000.)

muscle a striated appearance under a microscope. There are two types of muscle fibers: type 1, or slow twitch, and type 2, or fast twitch, fibers. Type 1 fibers are responsible for sustained contraction and, therefore, allow for endurance activities. Type 2 fibers have a faster contraction rate for a shorter duration than type 1 fibers and, therefore, produce more force at any contraction velocity.[1]

Skeletal muscle contraction occurs by the process of excitation–contraction coupling. This begins with acetylcholine release in the neuromuscular junction by a motor neuron with subsequent depolarization of the motor end plate. In response to this depolarization, voltage-gated calcium receptors on the sarcolemma undergo a conformational change which, due to direct mechanical linkage with the underlying sarcoplasmic reticulum receptor, causes a sharp release of calcium from the sarcoplasmic reticulum and subsequent muscle contraction via the sliding filament theory. According to this theory, the released calcium allows the thin actin filaments to be pulled by the thick myosin filaments in an adenosine tri-phosphate (ATP)-dependent cross-bridge cycling process that causes the filaments to slide along each other, resulting in sarcomere shortening and contraction. One axon can depolarize many myofibers called a motor unit. Motor units are recruited from smallest to largest for efficient contraction.[1]

The cross-sectional area of a healthy skeletal muscle is proportional to its capacity to generate a contractile force. The contraction velocity of muscle is a function of its fiber length. There are three main types of muscular contraction:

- Isotonic contraction: The muscle tension generated is constant because of the muscle length changing throughout movement.
- Isometric contraction: The muscle length remains constant while muscular tension is still produced.
- Isokinetic contraction: The total energy expenditure of the muscle remains constant while muscular length changes.

Isotonic and isokinetic contractions are a measure of dynamic strength, whereas isometric contractions are a measure of static strength.[1] These contractions are balanced by agonist and antagonist muscle groups that, although functionally oppose each other's actions, are necessary for proper movement and tension generation.[3]

Macroscopically, skeletal muscle has two junctions: a myotendinous junction and a bone–tendon junction. A myotendinous junction occurs where muscle transitions to tendon with continuous collagen fibers linking the two. A bone–tendon junction, or enthesis, refers to the tendons insertion to bone, which can be direct or indirect. Muscular strains and tears most often occur at the myotendinous junction because the maximum stress occurs here during an eccentric contraction, where the internal force is less than the external force.[1]

Joints

A joint refers to the space and connections made between the bones of the body that typically allow for relative movement. Joints are predominantly either diarthroses or synarthroses. Diarthroses, or synovial joints, allow for movement between bones, whereas synarthroses do not. The synovial joint can be further categorized by the type of movement it permits. The six groups in this categorization are a plane joint, ball and socket joint, hinge joint, pivot joint, condyloid joint, and saddle joint.[4]

The typical synovial joint consists of a synovial cavity between bones that is filled with synovial fluid and encased in a fibrous joint capsule. The articular surface is the boney end that is covered with approximately 2 to 4 mm of hyaline cartilage. Hyaline cartilage is composed of approximately 75% water, 15% type II collage, 10% proteoglycans, and 1% to 5% chondrocytes by mass. Hyaline cartilage is biphasic as it has both fluid and solid properties that function in load bearing.[2] Consequently, it functions to decrease the friction between the boney surfaces as well as to distribute the load. It further acts as a shock absorber by offloading compressive and shear forces at the joint surfaces. The absence of a direct neural and blood supply to articular cartilage limits its capacity to heal or regenerate. It is nourished by diffusion from two sources: synovial fluid and, to a lesser degree, through vessels within the subchondral bone. The lone cells of cartilage, chondrocytes, are mechanically stimulated and act to produce and maintain the integrity of the extracellular matrix.[1]

Further involved in friction reduction, shock absorption, and force offloading at the level of the joint is the viscous synovial fluid consisting primarily of hyaluronic acid. The synovial fluid is produced and maintained by the inner membrane layer of the joint capsule, referred to as the synovial membrane. There are two cell types in this layer: fibroblast synovial cells, which secrete the synovial fluid, and macrophage-like synovial cells, which impart limited immunity to the joint space. The outer joint capsule membrane, or fibrous membrane, is an avascular white fibrous tissue functioning to maintain the overall stability and alignment of the joint. Further adding to stability are extracapsular and intracapsular ligaments that articulate the ends of the bones and tendons inserting around the joint area to allow for movement of the joint.[1]

II. DEGENERATIVE CONDITIONS

Degenerative conditions of the musculoskeletal system are traditionally divided into either noninflammatory or inflammatory conditions despite "inflammation" being a pathologic hallmark of both. Noninflammatory typically refers to age- or trauma-related cartilaginous wear and tear, or osteoarthritis (OA), whereas inflammatory refers to autoimmune or metabolic etiologies of degeneration.[4]

Noninflammatory

OA is the most common arthritis and refers to age- or trauma-related degeneration of the articular cartilage with bone remodeling and formation. This nonuniform degeneration results in decreased shock absorption as well as increased frictional forces acting across the chondral surfaces of the joint, potentially exposing bone. As such, there will be secondary inflammation resulting in pain, stiffness, and swelling of the joint. Large weight-bearing joints, such as the knee and hip, are more commonly affected though any joint can be affected. Risk factors include advanced age, such that there is

X-ray evidence in at least 80% of people over the age of 55, female sex (2:1 to 3:1), obesity, history of trauma, and occupation (construction work, etc).[4] Age-related wear and tear OA without any other attributable causes is called primary, or idiopathic, OA. If a specific etiology can be attributed to the development of OA, it is considered secondary OA.

Patients will most commonly present with joint pain and swelling along with possible crepitus, decreased range of motion (ROM), and boney enlargement of the knee. They will often complain of morning stiffness that lasts less than 30 minutes as well as activity-associated pain that is relieved with rest. Labs such as complete blood count (CBC), erythrocyte sedimentation rate (ESR), and C-reactive protein (CRP) are typically within normal limits and are obtained to rule out any other possible etiologies. The hallmark radiograph findings of OA include decreased joint space, osteophytes, cysts, and subchondral sclerosis (Figure 1-4).

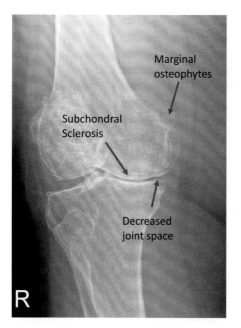

Figure 1-4 Right medial knee OA. Right medial knee demonstrating the hallmarks of OA as seen by decreased joint space, marginal osteophytes, and subchondral sclerosis.

Synovial fluid is noninflammatory with a WBC <2,000 per mm^3. The prognosis is dependent on the etiology, affected joint, and state of the articular cartilage.[4] The state of articular cartilage can be classified using either the Modified Outerbridge or the International Cartilage Repair Society grading scales. Both are graded from I to IV and stratify based on the thickness of the cartilage defect along with the exposure of subchondral bone (Table 1-1).[1]

Treatment is dependent on severity and extent of degeneration. Initial management should include weight loss along with physical therapy and exercise programs to strengthen the stabilizing muscles of the affected joint. First-line pharmacologic management in the form of nonsteroidal anti-inflammatory drugs (NSAIDs) for pain and inflammation with acetaminophen for pain as needed are then to be used.[4] Intra-articular joint injection can further be used in the event that pharmacologic management is not enough. Glucocorticoid

TABLE 1-1 Modified Outerbridge and International Cartilage Repair Society Cartilage Grading Scales

Grade	Modified Outerbridge	International Cartilage Repair Society
0	No defect	No defect
I	Chondral softening and swelling	Surface lesions consisting of superficial fissures and indentations
II	Partial-thickness defect not reaching subchondral bone	Partial-thickness defect involving <50% of cartilage thickness
III	Deep defect that extends to subchondral bone	Deep defect involving >50% of cartilage thickness to subchondral bone
IV	Full-thickness defect with complete exposure of subchondral bone	Full-thickness defect that penetrates subchondral bone

(steroid) with lidocaine injections is used to potently reduce the inflammation along with providing pain relief. These injections should be limited to no more than three to four times a year because overuse can accelerate joint degeneration. Hyaluronate injections are another option. These synthetic injections mimic synovial fluid and can restore some function and stability with subsequent pain control. If all of these measures fail to control the patient's pain and restore function, then surgery in the form of chondral transplants or joint replacement is indicated. If the patient is unable or not agreeable to surgery, then they should be referred to pain management.[5]

Inflammatory

Inflammatory degenerative conditions are a heterogeneous group of over 100 different forms of autoimmune or metabolic etiologies of disease that include rheumatoid arthritis, psoriatic arthritis, lupus, gout, etc. One of the most common autoimmune etiologies is rheumatoid arthritis (RA). RA is a systemic autoimmune disease that primarily attacks multiple joints, with 70% being the smaller joints of the hands, feet, and cervical spine. Here, immune over activity results in infiltration of synovial tissue with lymphocytes and plasma cells resulting in a persistent primary inflammation. Continued inflammation results in pannus, proliferative granulation tissue, that infiltrates and degrades articular cartilage along with the surrounding soft periarticular tendons, ligaments, and bursa and boney tissues. Other extra-articular manifestations of this disease include anorexia, lung fibrosis, renal amyloidosis, atherosclerosis, and anemia. Approximately 20% of patients will develop subcutaneous nodules.[4]

RA is present in about 3% of the US population with a mean age of diagnosis at 40, and female to male ratio of 3:1. Unlike OA, patients can commonly present with constitutional symptoms of fever and malaise. Further, in contrast to OA, patients will complain of morning stiffness and pain that lasts longer than 30 minutes and is improved with activity. Consequently, patients will further complain that the pain is worse at night with immobility. Like OA, patients will also have joint effusions. As this condition goes untreated, the persistent inflammation causes progressive damage to the periarticular and articular surfaces. The periarticular tendons will be prone to rupture, and common in the hands, patients will characteristically develop ulnar deviation, swan and boutonniere deformities (Figure 1-5). With continued cartilage and subchondral bone involvement, there is continued subluxation and dislocation of the small joints. RA tends to wax and wane, with flare-ups that must be acutely managed.[4] The development of new and targeted pharmacologic treatments has decreased the incidence of these long-term deformities.

Workup includes radiographic studies that will show surrounding soft-tissue changes, juxta-articular osteopenia, narrowing of joint space, and bone erosion along the joint margins. Laboratory studies include a CBC, ESR, CRP, as well as rheumatoid factor (RF) and anti-citrullinated protein antibody (ACPA) levels. RF is sensitive and not specific, whereas ACPAs have a specificity of approximately 95%. Synovial fluid is inflammatory with a WBC >2,000 mm^3. These historical, radiographic, and serum values can be used in conjunction with the 2010 ACR/EULAR Rheumatoid Arthritis Classification Criteria to establish a diagnosis. This classification system created a point value to a set of stratified clinical symptoms that include extent of joint involvement, serologic parameters, acute phase reactants, and duration to guide in establishing a diagnosis. A total score of 6 or more is sufficient for diagnosis.[4]

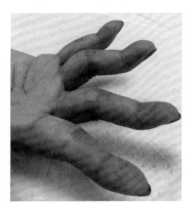

Figure 1-5 Clinical presentation of rheumatic hand with prominent swan neck deformities.

Treatment is primarily pharmacologic, aimed at inflammation and pain relief, as well as prevention of deformity and functional improvement. In patients diagnosed early with little systemic and joint pathologies, NSAIDs with or without oral steroids may be used for pain and inflammation. Prolonged and progressive disease, however, requires the use of immunosuppressive disease-modifying antirheumatic drugs (DMARDs), such as methotrexate, sulfasalazine, and leflunomide, which increase the risk of infection. If DMARDs are proven to be inefficacious after 3 months of use, biologic agents such as tumor necrosis alpha (TNF-α) inhibitors (eg, Infliximab), interleukin-1 inhibitors (eg, Anakinra), and targeted monoclonal antibodies (eg, Ritixumab) are used, albeit with an even further increased risk of infection. Surgery in the form of synovectomy and joint replacements are a last and not often sought out option.[6]

Gout is metabolic derangement resulting in an acute and inflammatory monoarthritis. More common in males, it is due to the precipitation of monosodium urate crystals in a joint. The underlying cause is either idiopathic under excretion of uric acid in about 90% of patients or the overproduction of uric acid in about 10% of patients. Patients will present with a swollen, red, and painful joint most commonly in the metatarsophalangeal (MTP) joint of the big toe (podagra). Synovial fluid will demonstrate negatively birefringent needle-shaped crystals under polarized light. Acute flare-ups are treated with NSAIDS, glucocorticoids, and colchicine. Preventative treatment thereafter centers around allopurinol to decrease uric acid levels.[7]

III. CONGENITAL CONDITIONS

Congenital orthopaedic disorders are predominantly the result of familial and genetic influences, though a few conditions can be attributed to maternal health and position in utero.

Skeletal Dysplasia (Osteochondrodysplasia)

Skeletal dysplasia, colloquially referred to as "dwarfism," is a broad term used to describe a group of over 350 different types of congenital developmental disorders of bone and cartilage, resulting in disproportionate short stature. The most common is achondroplasia with approximately 20% of cases inherited in an autosomal dominant manner and 80% of cases resulting from de novo mutations often associated with advanced paternal age. It is characterized by impaired cartilage proliferation at the growth plates because of an activating mutation of the fibroblast growth factor receptor. Consequently, these patients have impaired endochondral bone formation with normal intramembranous bone formation, resulting in shortened extremities disproportionate to normal sized head, chest, and trunk (Figure 1-6). Mental function, fertility, and life span

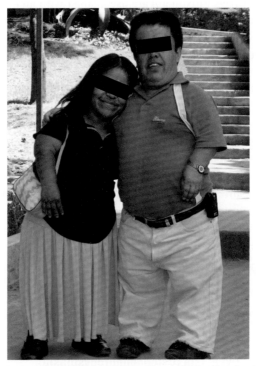

Figure 1-6 Patients with achondroplasia. Two patients with achondroplasia. Note the shortened extremities, which are disproportionate to normal-sized head, chest, and trunk. (Courtesy of Pablo Casteneda, MD.)

are not affected in achondroplasia. Treatment options are aimed at boosting the height of these patients. Somatotropin, a recombinant human growth hormone, can be initiated at 1 to 6 years of age for maximum benefit. Another option is an orthopaedic referral for limb lengthening surgeries using external fixators.[8]

Another common dysplasia is osteogenesis imperfecta (OI), a spectrum of disorders due to a qualitative and/or quantitative problem with type 1 collagen. There are nine types of OI with a variety of inheritance patterns and severity, though approximately 80% of cases are due to mutations of the COL1A1 or COL1A2 encoding type 1 collagen. Patients will present with blue sclera due to scleral lucency allowing the underlying veins to show through, along with growth retardation, osteoporosis, hearing loss, and dental problems. Patients are additionally further prone to repeat fractures, particularly during skeletal immaturity in childhood (Figure 1-7). To decrease the frequency and extent of fractures in these patients, bisphosphonates in conjunction with vitamin D

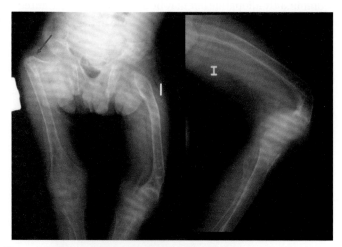

Figure 1-7 **OI femur fracture.** Femoral fracture secondary to OI. Note the diffuse osteopenia in this patient's radiograph along with evidence of previous fractures. Also note the malunited distal femur on the lateral view.

and calcium supplementation can be used. Possible orthopaedic interventions include osteotomy and intramedullary rodding for deformity correction and to allow properly aligned bone growth.[8]

Idiopathic/Syndromic/Metabolic

Clubfoot, or congenital talipes equinovarus, is the most common congenital orthopaedic condition, resulting in ankle and foot equinus, an adducted forefoot with a varus hindfoot (Figure 1-8). It is found in about 1/1,000 live births, is more common in boys with a 2:1 ratio, and approximately 50% of cases are bilateral.[7] It is most commonly idiopathic, though can be associated with arthrogryposis multiplex congenita and dwarfism. It is also associated with myelomeningocele as well as cerebral palsy due to gastrocnemius and tibialis posterior muscle spasticity. It is treated by either serial casting (Ponseti method) followed by a corrective brace for 2 years or by physical therapy and stretching (French method).[9]

Metatarsus adductus is another common condition that results in an adducted and inwardly angulated forefoot, or "in-toeing." It is predominantly idiopathic but may be associated with intrauterine positioning. Patients present with curvature in the lateral border

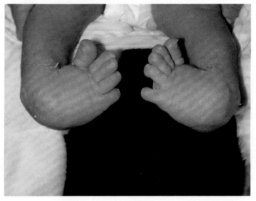

Figure 1-8 Clinical clubfoot. Clinical clubfoot as noted by the ankle and foot equinus, adducted forefoot, and varus hindfoot. (Courtesy of Pablo Casteneda, MD.)

of the foot instead of it being straight. As 90% of patients will improve without intervention, observation is indicated for the first 6 months of presentation. Persistence of the condition will require serial casting and/or subsequent bracing.[8]

Developmental dysplasia of the hip (DDH) is a spectrum of disease that encompasses etiologies from not of acetabular dysplasia to capsular laxity, resulting in subluxation/dislocation. Risk factors include female sex, firstborn child, positive family history for ligamentous laxity, and breech positioning. All children should be screened using the Ortolani test (dislocated hip relocated with elevation and abduction of the femur) as well as the Barlow test (adduction and depression of femur dislocates hip). If screening is positive, diagnosis should then be confirmed using ultrasound paying special attention to the alpha (angle between acetabular roof and ilium cortex) and beta (angle between ilium cortex and labral line) angles (Figure 1-9). Treatment depends on the etiology and severity of dysplasia and ranges from utilizing a Pavlik harness to corrective surgery.[8]

Congenital spinal deformities include congenital scoliosis and kyphosis. Both can be due to failures in segmentation, formation, or both (mixed). They are defects in formation in the 5th to 8th weeks' of gestation. Systemically, congenital scoliosis is associated with intraspinal, cardiac, or genitourinary abnormalities in a subset of patients. Most effective treatment is operative, though the exact options are controversial and range from a variety of fusions to resections.[1]

Rickets is a common metabolic condition that is characterized by a deficiency of vitamin D, calcium, or phosphorus, ultimately resulting

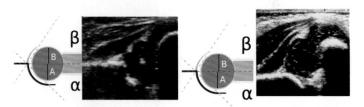

Figure 1-9 DDH ultrasound. Ultrasound evaluation and confirmation of DDH depicting α angle less than 60 and β angle greater than 55.

in poor bone formation. These deficiencies are most commonly dietary, but may also be the result of metabolic or malabsorptive defects. The primary effect is decreased osteoid mineralization, particularly at the metaphyseal growing ends of bones. Patients will present with failure to thrive, muscle weakness, and delayed teething as children. Frequently, adult patients will have repeat fractures, with angular deformity of the lower extremity, mostly commonly genu varum (Figure 1-10). Treatment is dependent on the etiology, which can be diagnosed based on a variety of serum markers.[8]

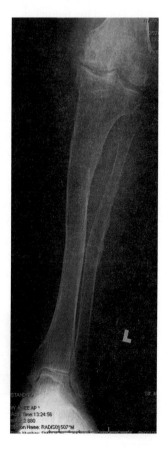

Figure 1-10 Rickets. Fifty-five–year-old female patient with rickets secondary to hypophosphatemia. Note the angular deformity and evidence of previous fractures.

IV. TRAUMATIC CONDITIONS

Traumatic care is a complex and interdisciplinary field that can require a multitude of differing practitioners for effective management. Orthopaedic traumatology is focused upon fracture care and is primarily noted by practitioners upon secondary and tertiary surveys. Noted fractures need to be reduced and immobilized.

Overall injury severity is dependent on the "energy" of impact. High-energy impacts, such as motor vehicle accidents, are more severe and associated with extensive soft tissue, vascular, and nerve damage. Low-energy impacts, such as tripping, do not have as extensive of soft-tissue damage. The physical examination signs of a fracture are listed in Table 1-2.[3] Most importantly, if there is abnormal movement secondary to fracture site movement or if there is crepitus between bone ends, it is a fracture until proven otherwise. Nonetheless, these signs can be absent or masked depending on the severity of the fracture pattern and anatomic location. When radiologically examining a patient for a suspected fracture, at least two views that are perpendicular to each other must be taken.[3] Once a fracture has been established, assessment of the 5Ps must be undertaken to rule out compartment syndrome.[1] These are:

1. Pain: Location, severity, and alleviating factors.
2. Pulse: Compare peripheral pulse distal to fracture with those on contralateral side to assess for vascular integrity.

TABLE 1-2	Fracture Physical Examination Signs
Fracture site movement resulting in irregular limb movement and impaired function	
Crepitus at fracture site	
Bruising, swelling, and point tenderness at site	
Pain with weight-bearing or physical stress	
Observable physical deformity	

3. Pallor: Color, temperature, and distal capillary refill for vascular integrity assessment.
4. Paresthesia: Assessment of sensation around fracture site and distal to it. Impaired sensation is an indicator of cell death.
5. Paralysis: Assessment of patient strength and mobility in affected limb.

There are three general phases to fracture healing starting with inflammation followed by repair and ending with remodeling (Figure 1-11). In all phases, bone blood flow is the factor with the largest impact on healing outcome.[1]

- Inflammatory phase: Characterized by hematoma formation and consequent granulation tissue formation. It is in this stage that osteoblasts and fibroblasts begin to proliferate to transition to the repair phase (Figure 1-11A, B).
- Repair phase: Refers to primary callus formation typically within the first 2 weeks of injury (Figure 1-11C, D). This soft callus

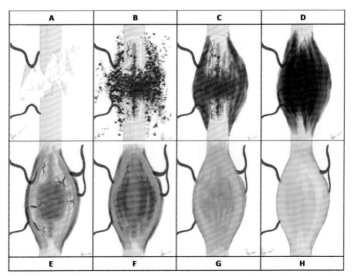

Figure 1-11 Phases of bone healing. A and B, Inflammatory phase. **C and D,** Early soft callus formation. E and F, Hard callus formation. **G and H,** Final bone remolding.

is eventually replaced by hard callus through endochondral ossification (Figure 1-11E, F). The exact mechanism of fracture healing at this phase is largely determined by the type of stabilization, if any.

- Bone remodeling: Initiates during the repair phase and continues years after fracture is clinically healed. This remodeling allows the immature bone of hard callus to be replaced with mature lamellar bone in a configuration and shape consistent with stress exposure, as stated by Wolff's law (Figure 1-11G, H).

Physiologic bone "healing" will occur with or without intervention. Fractures generally go on to union, but may have problems healing and result in one of three generic condition: delayed union, malunion, and nonunion. A delayed union heals properly with correct alignment, albeit slowly. A malunion results in union of the fracture ends, though with an improper alignment. A nonunion occurs when the healing of each of the fracture ends ensues separately and without union. The two extremes of nonunion are either hypertrophic or atrophic. A hypertrophic nonunion is one such that the fracture ends continue to proliferate and deposit bone in an attempt to make union with each other, but never do. An atrophic nonunion is the opposite wherein not enough bone is deposited at the fracture ends resulting in a "pencil-tip" appearance. Per Weber's classification, hypertrophic nonunions are considered "vascular" and are often the result of failed mechanical fixation, whereas atrophic nonunions are considered "avascular" and often the result of poor biologic healing (Figure 1-12). Long bones shaft fractures are more prone to nonunion. Healthy adult bone healing can take 6 to 8 weeks, whereas children's bones can heal as soon as 3 to 4 weeks.[3] It is the job of the Orthopaedic Surgeon to aid and direct the body's natural healing process in such a manner that proper alignment and mechanical stability are maintained.

Fractures are generally described and classified using the following terminology[10]:

- Open fracture: Bone penetrates through the skin and is exposed to outside contamination.

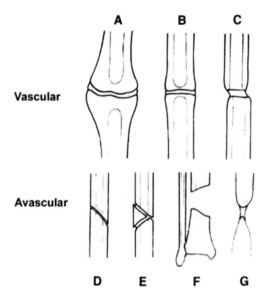

Figure 1-12 Weber's classification system of pseudoarthrosis.
Hypertrophic is at one extreme and considered to be a "vascular"
pseudoarthrosis, whereas atrophic is at the other extreme and considered
an "avascular" pseudoarthrosis. Vascular: A, Hypertrophic (elephant foot), B,
normotrophic (horse foot), C, Hypotrophic. Avascular: D, torsion wedge, E,
multifragmented, F, bone gap, G, Atrophic.

- Closed fracture: Fracture is confined within the body and does
  not break through the skin.
- Displaced fracture (Figure 1-13): Fractured bone segment not in
  correct alignment. Nondisplaced is in contrast.
- Stable fracture: The two bone ends are not likely to move relative
  to each other. An unstable fracture is in contrast.

Further description and classification is dependent on the
fracture patterns discussed as follows[10]:

- Transverse fracture (Figure 1-14): Fractured directly across
  the bone such that the fracture line is perpendicular to the
  bone's axis.

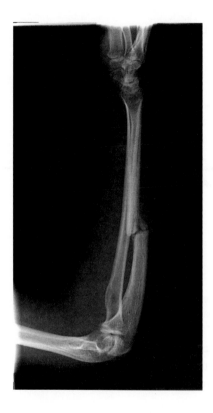

Figure 1-13 Displaced ulnar shaft fracture. Lateral radiograph of the forearm demonstration displaced ulnar shaft fracture.

- Oblique fracture (Figure 1-14): A fracture angulated approximately 30 degrees to the bone's axis.
- Spiral fracture: A twisting fracture around the bone secondary to excessive torsional forces.
- Comminuted fracture (Figure 1-14): A fracture that is fragmented in more than two pieces typically due to direct crushing trauma.
- Greenstick fracture: A buckling fracture such that one side of the bone has a compressed cortex, and the opposite side is curved and fractured. If the opposite side is curved and not fractured, it is called a buckled fracture. These two patterns are most common in children.

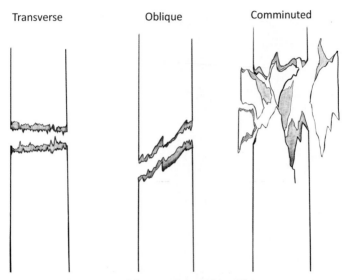

Figure 1-14 Transverse, oblique, and comminuted fracture patterns.
Depiction of transverse, oblique, and comminuted fracture patterns.

- Avulsion fracture: A fracture resulting from a boney fragment being torn away due to its ligamentous or tendinous attachments.
- Fatigue/stress fracture: Fracture secondary to minute, repetitive stresses over time.
- Pathologic fracture: Fractures secondary to osteoporosis, Paget's disease (Figure 1-15), tumors, cysts, and etcetera.

The majority of fractures are treated without surgery. Those that require surgery are generally treated with open or closed reductions and some type of internal or external fixation. Operative fracture management begins with debridement and decontamination of any open wounds, if present. Next, fracture reduction and subsequent immobilization help to properly create a suitable environment for fracture healing. Lastly, long-term rehabilitation of the limb must be established and maintained. The four primary methods of immobilization, in order of increasing invasiveness, are traction, external splinting or casting, external fixation, and

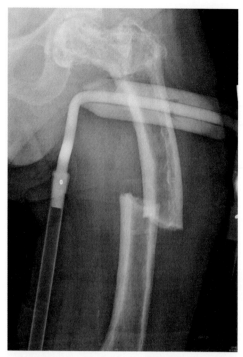

Figure 1-15 Pathologic Paget's fracture. Radiograph demonstrating pathologic fracture secondary to Paget's disease as evidenced by its "cotton wool" appearance.

internal fixation. If traction and/or splinting and casting are unable to immobilize the fracture in an acceptable position, then open reduction methods and external and internal fixation should be considered.[10]

- Traction: Mechanically manipulating limb in order to align fractured bone segments and regain initial stability (Figure 1-16). This is achieved via direct skeletal or skin/soft tissue traction as determined by fracture morphology and anatomic location.
- External splinting/casting: Externally maintain proper bone alignment. Casts provide rigid fixation, whereas splints do not.

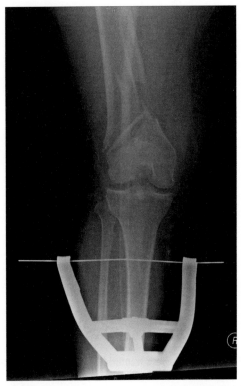

Figure 1-16 **Skeletal traction.** Anteroposterior (AP) radiograph of right femur and tibia demonstrating distal comminuted femoral fracture with trans-tibial skeletal traction.

- External fixation: A longer term external support consisting of pins that penetrate the skin to the bone providing proper alignment and mechanical stability of fracture ends. Carries a risk of infection.
- Internal fixation: Surgical intervention to properly reduce and permanently fixate fractures using hardware such as screws, plates, wires, and nails. Highest risk of infection.

Complications of fractures and fracture management, such as compartment syndrome, are discussed in Chapter 5 of this book.

V. INFECTIOUS CONDITIONS

Orthopaedic infections can be particularly devastating and infect everything from soft tissue (surgical site infection) to bone (osteomyelitis) to joints (septic arthritis) to implanted prostheses (periprosthetic joint infection). It is crucial to identify signs of infection early and treat accordingly. *Staphylococcus* and *Streptococcus* represent the majority of orthopaedic infections. Indeed, the *Staphylococcus* genus characterizes approximately 80% of orthopaedic infections. It is therefore prudent to empirically treat all presumed infections as such. Definitive treatment is best established based on the final culture and sensitivity profile of said culture.[1]

Acute Hematogenous Osteomyelitis

Acute hematogenous osteomyelitis refers to bacterial dissemination from the bloodstream to the bone. Children are more commonly affected than adults with particular localization to metaphyseal bone in the distal femur and proximal tibia. Vertebral osteomyelitis is the most common presentation in adults. Although *Staphylococcus aureus* is the most frequent pathogen, children under 3 can also be commonly affected by *Streptococci* and *Escherichia coli*. Patients typically present with the classic signs of infection including fever and general malaise along with localized redness, tenderness, swelling, heat, and loss of function of the affected limb with a reluctance to bear weight and pain unrelated to activity. Relevant labs include immediate blood cultures upon suspicion along with a CBC, CRP, and ESR. Acutely and early in the course of infection, the CBC may not reveal an elevated white count and an ESR can take several days to become elevated. CRP is typically elevated within 6 hours of inflammation and can be a particularly useful lab early in the course. The radiographic appearance instaed of radiography of osteomyelitis will be normal until about 2 weeks into the infection wherein elevation of the periosteum can be noted. An MRI, however, is sensitive and specific for osteomyelitis early on in the course and can further detail the extent of infection.[11]

Blood cultures should be taken immediately upon suspicion of this diagnosis followed by empiric intravenous administration of broad spectrum antibiotics until the cultures verify the pathogen. Empiric therapy should include vancomycin with gram-negative antibiotic, such as cefepime. The regimen should be subsequently adjusted based on the sensitivity profiles elucidated by the cultures. A falling WBC/ESR/CRP as well as a reduction of pain and the lack of fever following antibiotic administration is indicative of impending resolution and a good indicator to switch from IV to PO antibiotics. Total antibiotic administration typically lasts from 4 to 8 weeks.[12] Abscess development should be monitored. These signs include localized swelling, fluctuance, and persistent fever despite antibiotic administration. Surgical drainage will be necessary if these symptoms persist for 3 days. Complications include sepsis, septic arthritis, chronic osteomyelitis, and metastatic infection.[11]

Chronic Osteomyelitis

Chronic osteomyelitis (CO) most commonly results from incomplete or delayed treatment of acute osteomyelitis as well as from trauma; particularly open fractures. Risk factors for developing CO include diabetes mellitus, RA, smoking, immunosuppressing drugs including corticosteroids, and nutritional deficiencies. If stemming from a traumatic injury risk factors include extent of soft-tissue damage and contamination as well as vascular integrity such that the rate of infection increases with damaged arterial supply. *Staphylococci* are again the most common pathogen. Sickle cell anemia patients, however, are more likely to be infected by *Salmonella* as the etiology of their osteomyelitis.[12]

Patients may present with concomitant abscess formation and/or with draining sinus tracts. Patients with a previous fracture at the site can additionally present with a nonunion. They will commonly have an extended history of worsening pain, difficulty to weight bear affected area, and general malaise. Fever is usually absent and an elevated WCC, ESR, and CRP can be further indicative. Plain radiographs can demonstrate periosteal elevation and subperiosteal bone formation as well as areas of necrotic bone (sequestra) surrounded by new bone formation (involucrum).[1] MRI is the most sensitive and specific diagnostic tool for evaluating CO and further identifies any associated soft-tissue pathologies (Figure 1-17).

Unlike acute osteomyelitis, a biopsy or intraoperative sample should precede administration of empiric antibiotics, which must always be followed by surgical debridement for effective treatment. Debridement should remove all sources of infection including any dead or infected bone as well as the surrounding soft tissue. In the event of unstable or segmental loss of bone external fixation can be used to restore stability and encourage union. Local, eluting antibiotic therapies can also be applied at the site of infection.

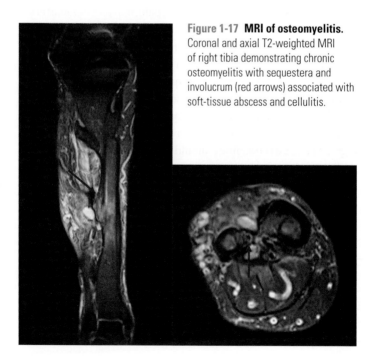

Figure 1-17 MRI of osteomyelitis. Coronal and axial T2-weighted MRI of right tibia demonstrating chronic osteomyelitis with sequestera and involucrum (red arrows) associated with soft-tissue abscess and cellulitis.

Complications include persistent or malunited fracture as well as squamous cell carcinoma from persistent inflammation.[11]

Acute Septic Arthritis

Acute septic arthritis (ASA) is a surgical emergency due to the rapidity with which it can destroy articular cartilage. Infection can be secondary to hematogenous spread, contiguous spread, or a penetrating trauma. *S. aureus* remains the most common causative pathogen overall. Infants can also become infected with group B *Streptococci*, and *S. pneumoniae* and *pyogenes* are not uncommon pathogens in older children. Infants are at particular risk as the entirety of their epiphysis is cartilaginous and susceptible to rapid destruction. Older children are at risk of avascular necrosis of the femoral head. *Neisseria gonorrhea* should be ruled out in sexually active adults.[11]

Patients typically present with fever, pain, malaise, monoarthritis with inability to weight bear the affected limb. Passive ROM will yield extreme pain with almost complete resistance. If the hip is affected, it is typically abducted in external rotation and slightly flexed. If the knee is affected, it is typical slightly flexed. Both joints should always be examined because the pain can be referred from either.[8] A WBC, ESR, and CRP should be obtained when ASA is suspected. Adults should undergo diagnostic aspiration as soon as possible, and the aspirate should be Gram stained and cultured with the appropriate sensitivity profile. A diagnosis of ASA is confirmed if bacteria are found on Gram stain or if there are greater than 50,000 WBCs/mL of aspirate without the presence of crystals. Suspected ASA in the pediatric population necessitates utilizing an algorithm to make the decision of whether or not to aspirate because of the high incidence of transient synovitis. There is a 95% probability if at least four of the following criteria are met: inability to weight bear, pyrexia over 38°C, ESR over 40, WBC over 12,000 per mm^3, and a CRP over 20. Empiric IV antibiotics should commence after aspiration, and surgical drainage should be performed as soon as possible.[11]

Periprosthetic Joint Infection

Infection secondary to arthroplasty can present early (within 3 weeks), late (after 3 weeks), or delayed and spread hematogenously from any other site. Infection presenting within 3 weeks or secondary to hematogenous spread presents and is treated in the same manner as septic arthritis discussed earlier.[11]

Late infection presenting 3 weeks after surgery is insidious in presentation and should not be missed. A history of postop would complications and poor pain control along with fever and an erythematous, swollen joint should prompt a diagnostic aspiration. If the hip joint is affected, an interventional radiologist should aspirate the joint under radiologic guidance. If confirmed, surgery to debride all affected tissue and remove any prosthetics is indicated, and intraoperative samples should be sent for assessment with antibiotic spacers implanted as a temporizing measure. A diagnosis is established from tissue cultures. Typically, a revision surgery is not undertaken until the infection fully subsides, indicated by normal serum inflammatory markers.[11]

REFERENCES

1. Miller MD, Thompson SR, Hart J. *Miller's Review of Orthopaedics.* Philadelphia, PA: Elsevier Health Sciences; 2015.
2. Einhorn TA, Buckwalter JA, O'Keefe RJ, eds. *Orthopaedic Basic Science: Foundations of Clinical Practice.* Rosemont, IL: American Academy of Orthopaedic; 2007.
3. Dandy DJ, Edwards DJ. *Essential Orthopaedics and Trauma.* Philadelphia, PA: Elsevier Health Sciences; 2009.
4. Iyer KM, ed. *General Principles of Orthopedics and Trauma.* Berlin, Germany: Springer Science & Business Media; 2012.
5. American College of Rheumatology Subcommittee on Osteoarthritis Guidelines. Recommendations for the medical management of osteoarthritis of the hip and knee: 2000 update. *Arthritis Rheum.* 2000;43:1905–1915.
6. Singh JA, Cameron C, Noorbaloochi S, Cullis T, Tucker M, Christensen R, et al. Risk of serious infection in biological treatment of patients with rheumatoid arthritis: a systematic review and meta-analysis. *Lancet.* 2015;386(9990):258–265.

7. Khanna D, Fitzgerald JD, Khanna PP, et al. 2012 American College of Rheumatology guidelines for management of gout. Part 1: systematic nonpharmacologic and pharmacologic therapeutic approaches to hyperuricemia. *Arthritis Care Res.* 2012;64(10):1431–1446.

8. Abdelgawad A, Naga O. *Pediatric Orthopedics: A Handbook for Primary Care Physcians.* Berlin, Germany: Springer Science & Business Media; 2014.

9. Su Y, Nan G. Manipulation and brace fixing for the treatment of congenital clubfoot in newborns and infants. *BMC Musculoskelet Disord.* 2014;15(1):363.

10. Egol KA, Koval KJ, Zuckerman JD. *Handbook of Fractures.* Philadelphia, PA: Lippincott Williams & Wilkins; 2010.

11. Clayton RA, Simpson AHR. Infection in orthopaedics. *Found Years.* 2008;4(8):309–313.

12. Calhoun JH, Manring MM. Adult osteomyelitis. *Infect Dis Clin.* 2005;19(4):765–786.

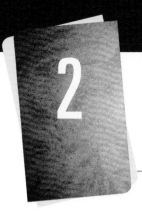

2

GETTING TO KNOW YOUR PATIENT

Stephanie C. Bazylewicz

I. INTRODUCTION

Although a thorough social history includes a routine set of questions that aid in getting to know a patient, it is important to look beyond a job title or a tobacco history to learn more about a patient's identity. Often as practitioners, we aim to solve an immediate problem, but it is important to first determine how patients' life will be affected first by their condition and second by each treatment option. Knowing this key information will help tailor the care they will receive to best suit their needs.

Because musculoskeletal conditions affect bones, joints, muscles, tendons, and ligaments, the majority of orthopaedic injuries and conditions inhibit motion and limit activity. First understand your patients' level of activity prior to the onset of their condition. Are they a high-performance athlete competing in marathons, competitive biking, or daily surfing? Are they a dedicated gym goer, yoga enthusiast, or martial arts student? How many miles do they run, jog, walk, bike, or swim on a weekly basis? What is the average level of intensity that they incorporate into their weight training routine? Are they sedentary, with little expectation beyond return to activities of daily living? In addition to setting patient expectations, this information may also help you diagnose their condition. Was the patient running five miles daily at a 10 minutes/mile pace but recently increased their routine to eight miles daily at a 9 minutes per mile pace? Increasing duration and intensity of activity abruptly may be the mechanism of injury in the development for a stress fracture for instance.

Not all patients will be high-performance athletes, but understanding their activity level is still significant to their treatment and recovery. Does your patient walk to work daily? If so, how many city blocks? Do they have to navigate stairs or a crowded area such as railway stations, bus stops, or subways? Would they be able to travel safely with a controlled ankle motion boot, cast, or sling in place, or while utilizing crutches, a knee walker, or a wheelchair? If the patient is not using public transportation, do they drive to work? Any time a patient is taking narcotic pain medication, muscle relaxants, or barbiturates, they must be advised against operating any moving vehicles or heavy machinery because of such side effects as sedation, drowsiness, muscle weakness, lightheadedness, and dizziness.

Other factors to consider regarding ability to drive include weight-bearing status, laterality of injury, injury-induced pain and/or postoperative pain, peripheral neuropathy, and joint stiffness. Further discussion with the patient is advised when lower extremity or spinal arthrodesis surgery is recommended because the loss of range of motion of the foot and ankle may impair ability to apply force to the brake pedal or accelerator, and the loss of range of motion at the level of the cervical spine can inhibit peripheral visibility while driving. One recommendation for all patients returning to driving is to start with a short drive in a traffic-free area and to be accompanied by another licensed driver. A companion is recommended in the event that driving exacerbates injury pain and the patient is not able to safely return home. Understand there is no "clearance" for driving. It is important to remember each patient has individual factors that will affect this recommendation and must be evaluated on a case-by-case basis. Table 2-1 provides general guidelines for return to driving after orthopaedic injury. Lower extremity impairment was evaluated as time required to perform an emergency stop. The above return to driving recommendations represent when braking function returned to normal. Upper extremity recommendations are based on ability to maneuver the wheel of the vehicle appropriately in situations where an abrupt swerve or sharp turn is necessary.

TABLE 2-1	Guidelines for Returning to Driving Based on Specific Injuries[1,2]
Injury/Surgery/Form of Immobilization	**May Return to Driving in. . .**
Major lower extremity fracture	6 weeks after initiation of weight bearing
Lower extremity fracture (diaphyseal)	12 weeks
Lower extremity fracture (periarticular)	18 weeks
Right total hip arthroplasty	4–6 weeks
Knee arthroscopy	4 weeks
Right knee ACL repair	4–6 weeks
Left knee ACL repair	2 weeks
Surgical repair of right ankle fracture	9 weeks
Bunion surgery	6 weeks
Cast, splint, or brace on right leg	Following removal of immobilization device
Upper extremity immobilization including elbow	Following removal of immobilization device
Forearm cast/splint	May be permissible while in place depending on fracture type

ACL, anterior cruciate ligament.

Although there are no state or federal laws restricting the operation of a motorized vehicle while wearing an immobilization device or during the postoperative period for an orthopaedic patient, the National Highway Traffic Safety Administration has published guidelines recommending the patient does not drive.[3] You may educate your patient that in the event of accident or injury, they may be considered liable if their disability prevented them from operating the vehicle efficiently. If the patient is diagnosed with a permanent disability, they can be referred to a driver rehabilitation specialist to determine if vehicle modifications can be made to allow safe driving. For those with temporary disability, physical and occupational therapists will be instrumental in rehabilitating the patient to safe driving function.

Now that you understand the patients' ability to navigate their world, determine what other activities of daily living will be affected by their injury. Do they reside in an apartment, condominium, or house? Are these dwellings multilevel? Do they live independently without assistance from friends or family members? Patients may also navigate stairs by sitting on the bottom or top stair, lifting their body up off the ground by pushing up off the ground, and navigating up or down to the next stair by pushing off with their uninjured lower extremity.

Does the patient shop for and prepare their own food? Will they be able to continue to prepare their own meals with their injury? If not, are take-out services available in their area and affordable to the patient? If the answer to these questions is not yes, the patient will require a home care assistance or visiting nurse services. Please refer to Chapter 9 section I for further information regarding home care services.

Inquire about hobbies and extracurricular activities the patient engages in often. Once you understand a patient's prior activity level, have a discussion regarding both their clinical and nonclinical goals following competition of treatment. This demonstrates your investment in their future and will help you set realistic expectations for treatment outcomes.

Hygiene: Do they bathe in a shower or a bathtub? Is there a handheld showerhead available? Postoperative patients should refrain from submerging and soaking incisions for 2 or more weeks following surgery to prevent wound maceration and dehiscence. Depending on the size and location of the incision, it may be acceptable to get the surgical area wet in the shower. Patients may wash with warm water and soap and blot or pat the incision dry following the shower. They should avoid scrubbing, rubbing, or abrading a healing wound. Likewise, they should avoid environments with high humidity and excessive sweating, whereas their incision is healing to prevent superficial soft-tissue infections.

If a cast or a splint is in place, patients must make a strong effort to keep the construct dry. Moisture will weaken the plaster or fiberglass material, therefore providing less support and stability to the healing bone or soft tissue. Padding that becomes damp may irritate skin and initiate soft-tissue infections. Several chain pharmacy stores stock waterproof cast covers or they can be purchased online (Figure 2-1). Patients often experiment with homemade versions, including plastic bags, trash bags, cellophane wrap, and tape. Do advise they apply several layers because a hole the size of a pin head will cause a leak significant enough to affect the cast or splint material.

Occupation: Understanding a patient's employment status goes well beyond if and when the patient will return to work. First determine if the patient is currently employed. If employed, is their employment status full time, part time, or per diem? If the patient is employed on a part-time or per diem basis, they may have more flexibility to attend office appointments, to attend physical or occupation therapy appointments, and to rest their injury. Those who are employed full time may need additional assistance in scheduling necessary appointments or complying with restrictions.

Next, what is the level of activity required by their job description? Must they stand or walk and if so, for how many hours per

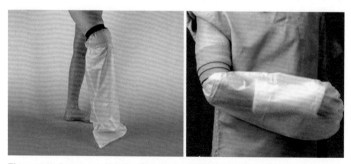

Figure 2-1 Lower and Upper Extremity Waterproof Cast Covers. Image demonstrating lower and upper extremity waterproof cast covers.

shift? Is there a lifting requirement, up to how many pounds, and how frequently must items be lifted? Do they have a more sedentary job where they may be seated for the duration of their shift? If their injury requires strict elevation of a lower extremity, can the accommodation be made by the employer? Does their job require significant typing, writing, or fine finger manipulation? If so, is their dominant extremity affected? Can job requirements be completed with an immobilization device in place and without jeopardizing healing ability?

If the patient is unable to return to work following a nonoperative injury or if surgery is indicated, have a discussion regarding timeline for recovery and when restrictions will be lifted. This will help the patient determine if they have adequate vacation or personal time to take off, or if they will need to apply for short- or long-term disability. Specific conditions may be treated appropriately with operative or nonoperative management. It is important to discuss the timeline of recovery for each of these options and to empower your patient with shared decision-making when determining the appropriate treatment option for them.

For patients who are unemployed and without health insurance, be mindful of the fact that office visits, therapy appointments, medications, immobilization or assistive devices, and hospital/surgical bills may be very expensive. Many hospitals will provide an estimate of expenses for a given surgery for self-pay patients. Be aware that specific services may be billed separately, such as a surgeon's fee, anesthesia fee, or hospital fee. Be sure to provide the patient with a comprehensive quote so there are no surprise bills following the surgery. Additionally, most institutions have a charity care service that patients may apply for. Case management teams and social workers are important resources to utilize when treating a patient in this financial category.

Do not be afraid to be creative in assisting a patient who may have limited access to services due to financial constraints. If there is space available in your office to store equipment, post a sign in the waiting room asking patients to donate crutches, knee walkers, slings, etc., once they have completed their rehabilitation. Pharmaceutical representatives will often drop off samples or financial assistance program packets to offices and hospitals. Do save these samples and financial assistance cards for those who are the most in need. Remember that even those with health insurance may have high co-pays for physical and occupational therapy appointments and may struggle with affording this fee. While formal therapy sessions are recommended, if the patient is unable to attend, physician-directed therapy is the next best option. Print off comprehensive home therapy instructions for patients targeting their specific injury. Examples of home therapy exercises can be found by searching exercise guides at http://orthoinfo.aaos .org. It is still recommended that the patient attend at least one session weekly to allow the therapist to assess their progress and adjust their therapy plan as needed. Make it a point to learn what services your specific hospital or practice offers so you are able to guide patients who need further assistance.

Lastly, determine if the patient's injury is work related. Please refer to Chapter 9 section III for further information regarding Worker's Compensation.

II. CULTURAL COMPETENCY

As trained medical professionals, physician assistants (PAs) have the privilege of caring for individuals with varying beliefs, values, customs, and knowledge from a variety of religious, ethnic, geographic, linguistic, and sexual backgrounds. The National Institutes of Health describes the importance of cultural competency as "critical to reducing health disparities and improving access to high-quality health care" and as "health care that is respectful of and responsive to the needs of diverse patients."[4] In studying cultural competency in the orthopaedic patient, Hussain et al. stated, "misinterpretation, uninformed assumptions, or stereotypical behavior may lead to anger and misunderstanding and can create obstacles to the administration of ethical, informed, and professional health care."[5] To maximize your ability to deliver high-quality health care to all individuals, familiarize yourself with the different cultures and religions that are prominent in your community.

The following are a few examples of disparities that have been identified in orthopaedics:

- In the Medicare population: African American patients have received 40% fewer total joint replacements including primary total hip arthroplasty and total knee arthroplasty (TKA) than white patients.[6] In the same study, it was found that the African American patients has a 24% higher 30-day readmission rate following TKA when compared with the white population.[6]

- A separate study utilizing an all-payer database found that "in comparison with whites (4.65/1,000 population/year), black (3.90), Hispanic (3.71), Asian (3.89), Native American (4.40), and mixed-race (3.69) populations had lower rates of total knee arthroplasty utilization."[7]

- In a study that evaluated disparities in hip fracture care "adjusting for patient and surgery characteristics, hospital/surgeon volume, social deprivation, and other variables, black patients were at greater risk for delayed surgery, reoperation, readmission, and 1-year mortality than white patients."[8]

- "A retrospective cohort study analyzed the pain management of 250 patients hospitalized for open reduction and internal fixation of limb fractures. Although there were no differences among racial or ethnic groups in nonopioid analgesics, white patients received significantly higher doses of opioid analgesics than did black and Hispanic patients. This racial and ethnic disparity in pain management persisted after controlling for operative time, comorbidities, number of procedures, length of hospital stay, and insurance status."[9]

These four examples alone demonstrate that race and ethnicity continue to drive the care patients receive today. Make it your goal to deliver culturally competent and ethical care to all patients you encounter.

III. BEHAVIORAL MEDICINE AND ORTHOPAEDICS

Remember that many orthopaedic conditions and injuries can be truly life changing to the patient and their families. They may abruptly create physical, emotional, and financial obstacles that patients and families need support in navigating. As such, treating orthopaedic conditions often requires a team of providers; do not overlook the mental health and behavioral professionals as part of the team. One study has demonstrated a strong association between depression and increased risk of complications, more specifically in the orthopaedic trauma patient.[10] Another study has indicated that nearly 40% of patients may have a preexisting psychiatric disorder, most commonly identified as depression in roughly 22% of patients and substance abuse in 17% of patients.[11] These preexisting conditions are compounded by the multifactorial stress from their new injury, delay or failure to administer psychiatric medications during their inpatient stay, and failure to receive instructions for psychiatric follow-up at their discharge.[11] Be vigilant for psychiatric conditions, both preexisting and new, in your patients and refer to the appropriate provider for early evaluation and treatment.

IV. BUILDING POSITIVE RAPPORT

Patients who associate a positive connection with and the ability to trust their provider will often show more compliant behavior with treatment recommendations. Make an attempt to be relatable. Try to factor into your visit time to discuss interest, hobbies, or family. A brief conversation regarding a common interest may help alleviate anxiety (Table 2-2).

Press Ganey is the leading provider in the United States for patient satisfaction surveys. It evaluates patient experiences, provider engagement, and clinical quality. In one study conducted by Etier et al. regarding patient satisfaction scores in an orthopaedic spine clinic, two variables were identified to alter the satisfaction score,[13]

TABLE 2-2	Do's and Don'ts for Building Positive Rapport[12]

Do	Don't
Help the patient to see you truly care for them	Make a patient feel rushed
Empower patients with shared decision-making; use a collaborative approach for all major decisions	Expect the patient to understand you if you have not taken the time to understand them
Contact patients who may seem to be having a difficult time physically or emotionally between appointments; more frequent communication will provide reassurance, relieve anxiety, and identify red flags	Have emotional or difficult conversations in a public area or an area with high background noise (hallways, cafeterias, and waiting rooms)
Be an active listener with an open posture and positive body language that maintains appropriate eye contact	Speak in highly technical terms or using medical jargon, instead use layman terms, draw pictures, use anatomy models for demonstration
Encourage patients to talk	Only deliver information regarding the immediate problem; remember the big picture
Respect cultural and religious beliefs	
Empathize with patient emotions	
Sustain dignity and maintain your patient's identity in all care that is provided	

one being pain and another being that the "provider spent enough time with you." When a patient answered that provider had spent enough time with them, the overall satisfaction score increased nearly 60%. As you gain more experience, you will begin to get a feel for those patients who require a few extra minutes to understand their diagnosis and review treatment options. Do spend this time with patients as it does significantly influence their health care experience.

Remember that you are not only the patients' health care provider but also their educator. A patient that fully understands their condition or injury is positioned to make educated decisions regarding treatment options. In addition to your conversation, provide the patient with literature or appropriate web sites to visit when they get home. This will help patients to avoid referencing less reliable sources and may reduce confusion by avoiding conflicting information. Lastly, try to anticipate your patients' needs. This will reassure the patient that you are invested in their health and well-being and will help build positive rapport.

REFERENCES

1. Marecek GS, Schafer MF. Driving After Orthopaedic Surgery. *J Am Acad Orthop Surg*. 2013;21(11):696-706.
2. Goodwin D, Baecher N, Pitta M, Letzelter J, Marcel J, Argintar E. Driving After Orthopedic Surgery. *Orthopedics*. 2013;36(6):469-474.
3. Physician's Guide to Assessing and Counseling Older Drivers. National Highway Traffic Safety Administration. http://www.nhtsa.gov/people/injury/olddrive/olderdriversbook/pages/Contents.html. Accessed March 20, 2016.
4. Cultural Respect. National Institutes of Health. https://www.nih.gov/institutes-nih/nih-office-director/office-communications-public-liaison/clear-communication/cultural-respect. Accessed July 14, 2016.
5. Hussain W, Hussain H, Hussain M, Hussain S, Attar S. Approaching the Muslim orthopaedic patient. *J Bone Joint Surg Am*. 2010;92(2):e2.
6. Singh JA, Lu X, Rosenthal GE, Ibrahim S, Cram P. Racial disparities in knee and hip total joint arthroplasty: an 18-year analysis of national Medicare data. *Ann Rheum Dis*. 2014;73(12):2107-2115.
7. Zhang W, Lyman SL, Boutin-Foster C. Racial and ethnic disparities in utilization rate, hospital volume, and perioperative outcomes after total knee arthroplasty. *J Bone Joint Surg Am*. 2016;98(15):1243-1252.

8. Dy CJ, Lane JM, Pan TJ, Parks ML, Lyman S. Racial and socioeconomic disparities in hip fracture care. *J Bone Joint Surg Am.* 2016;98(10):858-865.

9. Anderson KO, Green CR, Payne R. Racial and ethnic disparities in pain: causes and consequences of unequal care. *J Pain.* 2009;10(12):1187-1204.

10. McQueen M. Psychological distress and orthopaedic trauma: commentary on an article by Douglas S. Weinberg, MD, et al.: "Psychiatric Illness Is Common Among Patients with Orthopaedic Polytrauma and Is Linked with Poor Outcomes". *J Bone Joint Surg Am.* 2016;98(5):e19.

11. Weinberg DS, Narayanan AS, Boden KA, Breslin MA, Vallier HA. Psychiatric illness is common among patients with orthopaedic polytrauma and is linked with poor outcomes. *J Bone Joint Surg Am.* 2016;98(5):341-348.

12. Barkley PS. Building Rapport with your Patient: Positive Case Management Outcomes. National Association for Home care and Hospice. http://www.nahc.org/news/building-rapport-with-your-patient-positive-case-management-outcomes/. Accessed August 10, 2016.

13. Etier BE Jr, Orr SP, Antonetti J, Thomas SB, Theiss SM. Factors impacting Press Ganey patient satisfaction scores in orthopedic surgery spine clinic. *Spine J.* 2016;16(11):1285-1289.

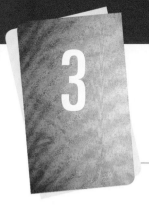

3

UNDERSTANDING YOUR ROLE IN THE PRACTICE

Stephanie C. Bazylewicz

I. ROLES AND RESPONSIBILITIES

Since the establishment of the physician assistant (PA) profession in the late 1960s, collaboration with a supervising physician and team-work have been cornerstones to a successful practice. Over the last 50 years, the practice model has increasingly granted greater autonomy to the PA by expanding beyond the traditional 1:1 pairing of PA to physician. Whether you are a new graduate or a well-experienced PA, it is important to learn the dynamic of how your prospective practice group functions. To understand your expected roles and responsibilities, it is helpful, when interviewing, to consider a few key questions and observations:

1. Is the practice a private practice with one, two, or more physicians? Is the position hospital based and specific to a group of physicians? Is the position service centered? Are there other practitioners including nurse practitioners and/or PAs in the practice, and, if so, how many? What is their level of experience, and how long have they been a part of this group? This information is important because aside from choosing orthopaedics as your specialty, it has been shown that physician support is one of the highest predictors of PA job satisfaction.[1] Understanding the size of the practice and current involvement and retention may reveal how much support you will receive as the newest addition to the team. It may also provide some insight into your working hours. Many service-based positions are set up as shift work, for example,

7:00 a.m. through 7:00 p.m., whereas assignment to a specific physician or group will often have general hour guidelines with flexibility to the end of your work shift. Remember, it is unlikely that another will be assuming your clinical responsibilities if you work for an independent physician or group. This often means you may need to remain at work until all high-priority assignments for that day are completed. If a more reliable and predictable schedule, a service-based, shift work position may be better suited for you as you can rely on being relieved at the end of your shift.

2. If you will be working with more than one physician, determine their individual expectations your availability for their specific practice. Have a group discussion with all parties involved regarding expectations for your time allocation. Request that each physician outline clinical and operative schedules and indicate where your skill can be utilized. Set up a transparent schedule that can be edited and viewed by all. Once you begin to work independently in the outpatient office or on the inpatient floors, you may require less segregation of your schedule. This will benefit each surgeon's practice by increasing your availability to their patients. In this model, you will offer outpatient appointments for each attending during the same office block.

3. Will your role in the practice be in the outpatient office, the operating room, and/or an inpatient hospital setting? If you will fulfill multiple roles, approximately what percentage of your time will be spent in each location? If there are multiple sites of practice (eg, surgery center, hospital-based operating room, outpatient offices), what is their proximity to each other, and how often will you commute among the sites?

4. Will orthopaedic residents or fellows have a permanent or temporary role in the practice? If so, will they be present in the outpatient office, rounding and managing inpatients, in the acute care clinic or emergency room, and/or assisting in the operating room? How will nonoperative clinical

responsibilities be divided? Other than the supervising physician, who is responsible for overseeing all duties? In the operating room, will the resident or fellow have priority as first assist or assume the role of lead surgeon? Is the practice volume sufficient for the PA to first assist in the operating room without compromising the learning opportunity residents and fellows? The setting of your position may determine the volume of residents and fellows present and their level of involvement in the practice. Most university teaching hospitals will have a larger volume of training physicians compared to more rural community-based hospitals. Although programs differ, institutions with an orthopaedic residency program or those that host residents annually may have less need for the PA in the operating room. If functioning as a first assist is a priority in your career, be sure to clarify this point prior to accepting a position. Please note that training physicians may be key resources to furthering your education as you train to become a skilled and experienced orthopaedic PA. Attending physicians are constantly educating young surgeons as a formal aspect of their training program. It is likely you will work as a team allowing you to absorb this information concurrently. Another perk of having training physicians at your institutions is that there will likely be cadaver labs, saw bones labs, morbidity and mortality lectures, and ongoing education lectures. If your schedule allows and you are permitted by the program director, attend these events and further your training too. **Helpful hint:** Many of these programs may be applied toward the continuing medical education (CME) hours that are required by the National Commission on Certification of Physician Assistants (NCCPA). With proper documentation, you can log these hours of education toward your recertification. Please see the section titled **Professional Expectations** for further detail.

5. Determine the level of additional support staff the practice? Is there a practice manager, a secretary, or a surgical scheduler?

Adequate support staff is necessary for a busy orthopaedic practice to run smoothly. Although the majority of your practice responsibilities will be clinical, PAs are often utilized to help off-load a significant amount of administrative responsibilities from the supervising physician. Establish protocols with the practice support staff for communications with patients, completion of FMLA, Worker's Compensation, No Fault Injury, disability paperwork, completion of prior authorizations, preoperative testing protocols, medication refills, and billing submissions. Many of these topics will be covered in detail in Chapters 9 and 10.

6. Does the practice have clinical support staff, including medical assistants, X-ray technicians, casting technicians, or physical/occupational therapists on site?

    1. Medical assistants: In the outpatient office, they may greet and escort patients to their examination rooms, document the chief complaint, medication history, allergies, and perform vital signs. In some practices, they will remove splints or casts upon instruction, gather procedure equipment, prepare injections, and apply prefabricated splints or devices. They may also prepare patient education handouts or gather discharge documentation.

    2. X-ray technician: Although most patients will require standard X-rays that the technician is trained to perform independently, some injuries require manipulation during imaging to acquire further information about the injury. One example is the ankle external rotation stress test that evaluates the syndesmotic and deep deltoid ligaments in patients with ankle fractures or high ankle sprains. A clinician other than the X-ray technician must be present to perform the manipulation. Again, establish routine protocols for specialized testing and order notations. Discuss with the technician if the X-ray should be performed with or without the cast or splint in place. Any modifications to standard orders should be communicated in person to avoid confusion and repeat imaging.

3. Casting technicians: Some practices will have technicians that specialize in the application of casts or splints. If you have this support in your practice, be sure to clarify the position of the extremity and all immobilized joints, which joints should be immobilized, which should have active range of motion, if a specific mold is required, and if postapplication imaging is necessary. Please see Chapter 7, section VI for further casting and splinting details.

4. Physical/occupational therapist: In-office therapists are an excellent asset to beginning the rehabilitation phase of a patient's recovery. They may perform an initial assessment followed by instruction and assistance with range of motion and strengthening exercises. They may also fabricate custom braces and facilitate scheduling the patient for the follow-up therapy sessions.

If these allied health professionals are not present in an orthopaedic practice, some of their roles and responsibilities may be transitioned to the PA. The following are a few key responsibilities that should be completed before the end of any clinical day to provide excellent orthopaedic care and to promote good office practice.

1. Complete all patient-oriented documentation, including admission history and physical examinations, inpatient progress notes, discharge notes, outpatient new and established patient notes, and procedural notes (Of course this assumes you have completed outpatient office hours and rounds on all inpatients.)

2. Return patient and health care provider secure messages and phone calls.

3. Proactively call all discharged postoperative day 1 patients for follow-up, to answer any questions and to clarify postoperative instructions.

4. Complete medication refill requests and visiting nurse/therapist orders.

5. Complete pending prior authorizations and peer-to-peer evaluations.

6. Complete all administrative paperwork, including FMLA, WC, NFI, and disability paperwork.
7. Submit all surgical and clinical billing documentation.
8. Review surgical clearances for upcoming operations. Confirm cardiac, pulmonary, and medical clearance as well as whether the blood type and screen/cross are present in the patients' chart if necessary. Verify preoperative images necessary for surgery are accessible or that the patient has been reminded to bring their films on the day of surgery.
9. Preorder imaging for patients who require routine postoperative imaging for upcoming follow-up appointments.
10. Complete any assigned institutional education.
11. At the end of the day, contact your supervising physician and support staff to verify that there are no outstanding tasks requiring completion at this time.

Create a checklist similar to the list above with responsibilities specific to your practice. Review your checklist at the end of each day to ensure you have been thorough in fulfilling your role in the practice.

II. GOALS AND EXPECTATIONS

If you are a new graduate or an experienced PA in another specialty, begin your orthopaedic career by setting realistic monthly goals in addition to overall goals for your first 6 months and first year in practice. By establishing goals, you will create guidelines to achieving success. Ask your supervising physician to collaborate with you. Their input will assist in prioritizing what may seem like an initially daunting tasking. For the experienced orthopaedic PA who may be familiar with extremity anatomy, know fracture classifications and understand operative indications, your focus may be on streamlining your workflow, optimizing patient experiences and outcomes, and educating the next generation of orthopaedic clinicians. When developing your goals, incorporate the SMART

TABLE 3-1	SMART Goals

Specific: Who? What?
Measurable: Answers the question how?
Attainable: Goals are reasonable and realistic to achieve.
Results Oriented: Goals are aligned with your mission and focused.
Time-bound: Set a deadline.

goal setting strategy to help create realistic and achievable goals (Table 3-1).[2]

Consider the following listed topics as possible areas of focus when defining your goals. Although it is important to develop your clinical and operative skill set, you may also be interested in advocating for the PA career or mentoring future and current PA students.

Physician Assistant Goal Setting Topic List

1. Broadening orthopaedic and medical knowledge: fracture classifications, operative and nonoperative indications, preoperative workup, osteoporosis workup, oncology workup, laboratory testing indications and interpretation, pathophysiology of bone metabolism, commonly used medication and their indications, side effects and dosing, weight-bearing statuses and indications, X-ray, ultrasound, MRI, CT, bone scan and DEXA scan indications and interpretation, orthopaedic assistive devices, patient education, and development of physical and occupational therapy protocols.
2. Proficiency at bedside procedural skills: closed reduction of fracture/dislocations, application of skeletal traction, casting and splinting including windowing and bone stimulator application, brace application, incision and drainage, therapeutic injections, joint/cyst aspirations, administration of local anesthetic, wound closure, suture and staple removal, in-office wound debridement, application and removal of negative

pressure wound therapy devices and drains, compartment pressure measurement, and external fixation frame adjustments.

3. Proficiency as a first assist (if applicable): positioning and preparation of the patient, anatomy, knowledge of instrumentation and implants, obtaining and maintaining exposure, preparing grafts, application of internal devices, deep and superficial wound closure, postoperative prescription and discharge instructions, discharge examination.

Remember that although you have likely had one or two operative rotations as a student, there are thousands of tools, instruments, and implants that you will begin to use regularly in the orthopaedic operating room. Many of these will be new to you. Start by learning the basic instruments you will use regardless of the surgery being performed. Next determine the 3, 5, or 10 surgeries that are most commonly performed by the surgeon. Although each surgery will be unique and specific to the patient, many routine surgeries such as anterior cruciate ligament repairs, rotator cuff repairs, and carpal tunnel releases will have steps that you repeat each time the surgery is performed. Learning the routine steps for common surgeries will allow cases to move along more fluidly and without hesitation.

4. Excellence in nonoperative practice: maximizing efficiency and availability in the outpatient office, decreasing wait time, streamlining work flow, providing patient education materials, prompt completion of prior authorizations, billing submission and documentation.
5. Teaching: mentoring PA student candidates and current PA students, lecturing, supervising, and instructing skills labs.
6. Academic research and publishing.
7. Attending and presenting at academic conferences.
8. CME, supplementary courses, and certifications: ACLS, BLS, PALS, NRP, central line placement and/or ultrasound guidance, thoracotomy tube placement, and infection certification.

9. Networking with other PAs and health care professionals: resources at AAPA.com connect and attending AAPA annual conference, LinkedIn, social media, blogging, alumni events at alma mater, establishing relationships with referring physicians, primary care physicians, radiologists, pharmacists, physical and occupational therapists, and imaging technicians.[3]
10. Volunteerism and community outreach.
11. Work–life balance: maintain hobbies and outside interests, cultivating personal and professional relationships.
12. Professionalism and ethics: integrating ethical and moral behavior, expressing empathy and intellectual honesty.

After you have established goals and benchmarks for yourself, create a system for evaluation of proficiency. Your supervising physician will be an integral player in helping you to achieve these goals, evaluating your ability and encouraging you to continue to grow as a PA. Aim to continually reassess your progress and understand that some skills will take more time to achieve proficiency in than others. Understand your limitations and do not feel embarrassed or ashamed to ask for assistance or supervision. Until you feel confident completing a procedure or attending to patients independently, all parties involved including the patient, your supervising physician, and you will appreciate your recognition of limitations. Do not forget your oath to nonmaleficence: first, do no harm. If you remain focused and eager to learn, with in time you will gain the knowledge and skill to work efficiently with confidence.

Professional Expectations

In a survey of practicing orthopaedic surgeons, the ability to work independently, to express accurate and timely communication, and to be reliable were commonly identified expectations for PAs. Ability to work independently can be defined as having the education, experience, and aptitude to take a thorough history and perform a physical examination which allows the PA to formulate a diagnosis and treatment plan. Regarding procedures, the PA should be assessed for the ability to perform the procedure safely and competently and to have the skill and knowledge to appropriately handle any complication resulting from the procedure. Often you will hear an attending say, "See one, do one, teach one." Although you may feel confident you can perform the skill after completing two procedures, many hospitals require supervision of 10 proficiently completed procedures prior to granting you privileges. Your supervising physician will determine when you have met these criteria. It is unlikely that you will work independently immediately after beginning your position. Have a discussion with your attending to set expectations for meeting this benchmark. If you are a new graduate, it may take between 3 and 6 months before you have accumulated enough experience to feel confident assessing and treating patients without someone checking your work in real time. Most importantly, know your limitations and when to ask for help.

Accurate and timely communication is crucial to providing high-quality patient care. In a study conducted by Lundine et al., skillful communication was more commonly defined as accurate and appropriate use of language, that is, content versus process, (how it was said).[4] Your communications will be divided into two major categories: the first classification concerns your interactions with patients and their families, and the second concerns your interactions with other members of the patients' health care team including your supervising physician. With your patient, the accurate and empathetic communication of information will aid in building a strong rapport. Time and fatigue have been identified as two major barriers to effective communication. Spending an adequate amount of time with a patient can be directly translated into patient satisfaction and inversely correlates with number of malpractice suits.[5] Before leaving any examination room, use the phrase, "Do you have any further questions or concerns that I can address?" and/or "Do you understand everything we have talked about?" These types of questions empower your patient to clear up any confusion and to leave your interaction feeling fulfilled.

Regarding timeliness, set the patient's expectation for future communications appropriately. If you state that you will be in touch within 2 to 3 days following the completion of a laboratory test, do follow through on your word. Remember some patients may feel anxious about testing results and delayed communication may amplify this feeling. Use similar language when concluding a telephone encounter and remind the patient that if they have further concerns, scheduling an appointment to discuss such matters in person may be more beneficial.

Most importantly, be sure to always convey the same message you feel your attending would. This is especially important early on because you are still learning their preferences and operative versus nonoperative indications. If in any way you are unsure of the diagnosis or treatment plan, it is best to limit the information you pass along to the patient and reassure them that the surgeon will cover these topics. Additionally, communication with your attending should be accurate and prompt. Communicating findings of a physical examination and current level of activity is particularly important as these often impact the treatment plan. Learn the appropriate format of presenting a patient and with time modify your presentation to the surgeons' preferences.

Example of patient presentation: Mr John Smith is a 57-year-old Caucasian male with no significant past medical history presenting to clinic for 6-week postoperative tibial plateau open reduction internal fixation follow-up. He reports erythema surrounding his incision site ×3 days. He denies fevers, chills, drainage from incision, and change in level of discomfort. He is afebrile, and vitals are within normal limits. His physical examination reveals that the wound is well healed, clean, dry, and intact with 3 × 4 cm area of erythema at the inferior aspect of the incision. I assess that the patient has developed a superficial cellulitis and I will begin him on a course of Keflex. He will follow up in 1 week to assess for resolution in the condition.

This presentation indicates to your attending **who** the patient is, what he was **initially treated** for, what his **current complaint** is, your **assessment**, **diagnosis**, and **treatment** plan. Lastly, escalate pertinent information to your supervising physician promptly. Situations requiring prompt attention include risk of life or limb, operative and nonoperative complications, delayed healing, dissatisfaction with care, noncompliance with treatment protocol, narcotic abuse, etc. The more time you spend at a particular practice, the better you will understand the style of communication your supervising physician prefers and what works best for your team.

Lastly, surgeons highly value reliability in a PA. How can you become a truly reliable PA? To start, arrive at the operating room and to office hours 15 to 30 minutes prior to the official start time. This will allow you time to gather equipment necessary for positioning your first patient, seeing the patient in the preoperative holding area, and dispelling any concerns while answering last minute questions, preparing or obtaining procedure consent, smoothing over any last minute hiccups with surgical clearance, pregnancy testing, morning of type and screen/cross, anesthesia questions/concerns, and preparing preoperative imaging needed to begin the case. In the office, you may prepare operative booking packets, evaluate who will likely need imaging at their appointment, and review your schedule for patients who may need additional attention. Some flexibility is required unless working for a service where at the end of your shift, you are being relieved by another PA. An accurate handoff of information is critical. Be sure you are available for another 30+ minutes following the completion of your day to complete any documentation, paperwork, prescribing, return patient calls, and prepare for the following day. If you have outside commitments that may infringe on working hours, be sure to inform your supervising physician as early as possible so necessary accommodations can be made.

Reliability is not just showing up on time and when needed but also being able to perform an accurate, thorough, and reproducible history and physical examination with special attention given to the neurovascular examination. Often there are key aspects of the history and physical, which unfortunately can easily be neglected in a busy practice but are essential to high-quality orthopaedic care. Additionally, thorough evaluation of imaging and knowledge of when advanced imaging is indicated are essential to successfully diagnose all orthopaedic conditions. Be assured that you are working as part of a team, and when unsure of how to proceed with the workup, diagnosis, or treatment, the best approach is to ask for help.

Additional aspects that determine your reliability include always representing the practice and the surgeon in a professional manner that is in line with the mission and goals established by the institution. This includes appropriate dress, language, cleanliness, and respectfulness toward patients and coworkers. It also means arriving at work, ready to work, with a positive attitude and without distractions. If assigned ongoing recurring assignments, do complete them as expected and without periodic reminders by your supervising physician. You may utilize the recurring features of an electronic calendar for reminders if necessary. Other prioritized expectations identified by orthopaedic surgeons include the desire to care for patients, integrity, and motivation to continue learning. Find out your attending physician's expectations for your position early on. The more aware you are of the role they hope for you to fulfill, the easier it will be for you to succeed in your practice.

Professional expectations also include maintaining all license and certifications without lapse in privilege. The NCCPA now certifies all PAs with a passing score on the PANCE for 10 years. PAs are required to then take and pass the PANRE in the 9th or 10th year of their certification to maintain their privileges. To schedule the PANRE, an online application must be submitted and US$350 payment processed. The PA then has 180 days to take the examination once registered. Although 60% of the PANRE will be a generalized examination similar to the PANCE, you may choose the content of the remaining 40% to be concentrated in adult medicine, primary care, or surgery. Further questions regarding the PANRE may be addressed at http://www.nccpa.net/faq#practice-focusedpanre.

In addition to passing the PANCE and PANRE, every 2 years PAs are required to engage in 100 hours of CME and to pay a certification maintenance fee of US$130. Fifty of these CME hours must be classified as Category I credits. Category I credits can be earned by completing preapproved certification programs listed at http://www.nccpa.net/cme-preapproved. Other Category I credits are earned by engaging in activities approved by one of the following organizations: AMA, AAPA, AAFP, AOA, RCPSC, CFPC, or PACCC. Documentation that the course was approved by one of these organizations and proof of completion must be kept for 2 years following each CME earning window in case of an audit. The remaining 50 credits may be classified as Category I or II credits. Category II credits are defined as "any medically related activity that enhances the role of a PA (including journal reading)" per the NCCPA. There is no limit on quantity of hours logged in a specific activity for Category II CME, and there is no formal audit process for Category II education.

Maintaining your license will vary on a state-by-state basis. Please refer to your state licensing board for further information. Often, to maintain a license, a simple demographic form and fee need to be paid and submitted prior to your current license expiring. Most states issue licenses for 3-year periods. Some states do require certain certifications to maintain licensure such as infection control and barrier precautions certificates.

Other certifications such as ACLS, BLS, and PALS should be renewed every 2 years to maintain proficiency in such skills. DEA licenses also need to be renewed every 3 years by completing the form at https://apps.deadiversion.usdoj.gov/webforms/jsp/regapps/common/renewalAppLogin.jsp. In addition to these state-specific and national license and certification maintenance expectations, your employer may also require institution-specific continuing education modules. Often this includes education regarding fire safety, evacuation procedures, code status and disaster protocol, blood borne pathogens, and human resource protocols. It is expected that you complete this education in a timely fashion. Often this education is repeated on an annual basis. Additional compliance measures include TB testing, respirator fit testing, influenza vaccination, and an annual employee physical.

Personal Expectations

Just as your employer and supervising physician have expectations regarding your performance and ability as a PA, you too should have expectations of them. Most critical to your professional development is the support and training you receive from your supervising physician. Recall the PA Goal Setting Topic List on page XXX. Items 1 through 3 list many of the procedural skills and medical topics that you must master. Request a 30- to 60-minute weekly session that is protected time dedicated to covering one of these topics in depth. If a physician is established, they will likely have developed preferences for a variety of aspects of their practice, such as workup protocols, physician referrals, casting and splinting material, style of application, devices used, etc.

An example of an osteoporosis workup review: First obtain history of menarche, menopause, number of pregnancies, abnormalities in menstrual cycle, previous fractures sustained and mechanism of action, diet, involvement in weight-bearing exercises, family history of osteoporosis/osteopenia, tobacco history, use of corticosteroid, barbiturate, or thyroid medications, prior lab study results, prior DEXA scan results, and prior medication therapy if previously diagnosed with osteoporosis. Next, if labs have not been completed in the last 3 to 6 months, order calcium and 25-hydroxyvitamin D levels. A reference range for normal calcium levels is 8.6 to 10.2 mg/dL. Vitamin D deficiency is defined as 25-hydroxyvitamin D blood level <20 ng/mL, and vitamin D insufficiency is defined as a level between 21 and 29 ng/mL. Next, is a DEXA scan indicated? If so, interpretation of results is as follows: normal bone density, T-score $>$ -1; osteopenia, T-score between -1 and -2.5; osteoporosis, T-score below -2.5. When is a rheumatology or endocrinology referral recommended? Does the practice have preferred providers?

If not referring to another provider for management of osteoporosis or osteopenia, what are the preferred doses of calcium and vitamin D supplementation? What other medications are available to treat osteoporosis? What other topics should be covered during patient education? After reviewing osteoporosis with your supervising physician, spend the next week reading the literature regarding diagnosis and treatment recommendations.

Not only may you expect formal training from your supervising physician, but it is necessary to have open lines of communication during all working hours. If a physician is not on-site, you must have a guaranteed method of contact. Will they be available via phone call, secured e-mail, or text messaging with the ability to respond to you promptly? Establish expectations early to avoid poor communication and prevent compromising patient care.

Other expectations you may have of your supervising physician include the respect for your personal time, ease in your ability to request time off promoting work–life balance, on-site ongoing education and clinical support, a positive attitude, a pleasant working environment, a safe and code-compliant working facility, instrumentation, materials, and support staff necessary to provide excellent patient care, targets for increase in salary with excellent performance, allotment of CME time and financing, malpractice insurance, and a confidential incident reporting system. As there are countless other expectations you may have of your employer, be sure to communicate your needs early and often to ensure that your goals are aligned for a successful practice.

REFERENCES

1. Hooker RS, Kuilman L, Everett CM. Physician assistant job satisfaction: a narrative review of empirical research. *J Physician Assist Educ.* 2015;26(4)176-186.
2. Professional Goal Setting for PAs. Blog of a Canadian PA. Available at https://anneccpa.wordpress.com/2012/12/26/professional-goal-setting-for-pas. Accessed March 20, 2016.

3. American Academy of Physician Assistants. Frequently asked questions: Optimal team practice—new policy adopted by AAPA in May 2017. https://news-center.aapa.org/wp-content/uploads/sites/2/2017/05/OTP_FAQ_FINAL.pdf. Accessed August 14, 2017.

4. Lundine K, Buckley R, Hutchison C, Lockyer J. Communication skills training in orthopaedics. *J Bone Joint Surg Am*. 2008;90(6):1393-1400.

5. Adamson TE, Bunch WH, Baldwin DC Jr, Oppenberg A. The virtuous orthopaedist has fewer malpractice suits. *Clin Orthop Relat Res*. 2000;378:104-109.

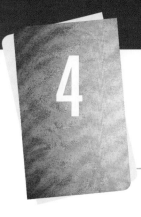

4

EVALUATION OF THE NEW PATIENT

Stephanie C. Bazylewicz and Gabrielle C. McIntyre

I. INTRODUCTION

Design your greeting and introduction. What does this entail? Typically, this includes a welcome greeting, your name, who your supervising physician is, and your position. A handshake and a warm smile go a long way toward establishing a positive rapport immediately. For example, "Hello! Welcome to our office. My name is . . . and I am Dr. . . .'s physician assistant (PA)."

Although the profession of PA has been established for nearly 50 years, and there are more than 130,000 certified PAs in the United States, many patients, or accompanying family or friends, will commonly ask you, "What is a PA?"[1] Be able to concisely answer this question while instilling confidence in your patient that you are their advocate and part of their health care team. For example, "A PA is a licensed and certified practitioner that works in conjunction with a supervising physician. Today, Dr. . . . and I will be working together to answer your questions and address your concerns, and I am here to get things started."

Do not be surprised, or offended, if the response is, "So why didn't you study for a few more years to become a doctor?" or "So when will you become a doctor?" Be proud of your profession and respond politely. Despite having this conversation, patients often are unsure of how to address you and may say, "Doctor . . . ." By law it is your obligation to be sure the patient understands you are not a doctor. You may gently reiterate this point but recommending they refer to you by your first name or full name without a title.

This is a good opportunity to determine how the patient would like to be addressed as well. Some patients feel strongly about being addressed formally as Dr., Mr., Mrs., or Ms., just as others may be adamant about being addressed by their first name. Never use terms like "dear" or "sweetie." Next, if there are any visitors present in the room, ask what the relationship is between the patient and the present parties. Do not assume. For example, "Please tell me how are you two related?" Once the relationship is established, and if the patient is 18 years or older, ask if they are comfortable moving forward with a history and physical with others present in the room. Do not forget, a parent or guardian must accompany all minors.

If a patient is not English speaking, be sure to use an interpreter for the encounter. Avoid having family members or friends translate because key information may be lost in the translation or opinions other than the patients are interjected. Include the translator's identification number in your official documentation.

In some situations, a patient will be brought in by emergency medical services or an ancillary service from a rehabilitation center or a nursing home. Always address the patient directly and determine their capacity for providing a history. The home institution will likely send paperwork that includes a current medication list and an additional sheet for orders and visit updates. If the patient is unable to communicate their history, contact the home institution and speak with the patient's primary care physician or nurse. As a last resort, the transport team may be able to provide information.

Once you have covered all the above, segue into the history and physical with an open-ended statement. For example, "Please tell me what brings you in to the office today."

II. HISTORY

During this portion of the patient encounter, you will collect subjective data. Must cover topics include chief complaint, past medical history, past surgical history, family history, social history, current medications, and allergies to drugs or foods.

The Chief Complaint

This is the patient's reason for seeking care. Once they have explained the reason for their visit, further characterize the complaint by determining the history of the present illness. Begin with onset of symptoms: acute vs. gradual, and length of time symptoms have been present. Was there an inciting event and if so what was the mechanism of injury? Next, determine if there are any palliative or provocative factors. Palliative factors may include: rest, medication, heat, ice, physical or occupation therapy, injections, bracing devices, position/posturing, or previous surgical intervention. Provocative factors may include: repetitive motion, position/posturing, range of motion, resistive movements, and ambulation. Next determine the quality and characteristics of symptoms: if the complaint is pain, is it sharp, dull, aching, or burning? What is the region the symptoms are located in, and do they radiate to another location? What is the severity of symptoms? You may use a 1 to 10 scale to quantify severity. What is the timing of symptoms and are they constant, intermittent, or progressive? The chief complaint may include symptoms such as pain, weakness, stiffness/loss of range of motion, instability, numbness, and tingling.

Past Medical History

First, begin with the patient's pertinent past medical history. This includes diagnoses that may cause the chief complaint, may have the chief complaint as a symptom, or may make the patient susceptible to their specific injury or condition. For conditions identified, learn the details of onset, diagnosis, treatment to date, and complications.

Next, review the patient's complete past medical history. This includes all chronic conditions and hospitalizations to be documented in reverse chronologic order. For conditions where laboratory assessments or diagnostic evaluations were likely performed, you may request their most recent testing results.

- Common childhood illnesses: Asthma, measles, mumps, rubella, chickenpox, pertussis, rheumatic fever, recurrent ear infections.

- Common adult illnesses: Hypertension, coronary artery disease, diabetes, high cholesterol, cerebral vascular accident, myocardial infarction, asthma, COPD, thyroid disease, renal disease, seizures, cancer, anemia, substance abuse, depression, and anxiety.
- Common screening tests: Dual-energy X-ray absorptiometry (DEXA) scan, hemoccult, lipid panel, and metabolic panels.

Past Surgical History

It is important to document details of all prior surgeries. This includes: surgery performed, date of surgery, location of surgery (hospital name and city), surgeon, and indication for surgery as well as any adverse reactions to anesthesia. If relevant, limb and laterality and presence of an implant should be recorded. Note any prior adverse effects to anesthesia and severity of the effect.

Family History

Begin this section of history with an open-ended question such as, "Has anyone in your family had a similar condition or symptoms?" This will allow the patient to discuss past family history pertinent to orthopaedics. Documentation should also include major systemic conditions including: rheumatoid arthritis, osteoarthritis, hypertension, diabetes, high cholesterol, cerebral vascular accident, myocardial infarction, coronary artery disease, cancer, hematology/clotting conditions, etc. A thorough history will include three generations of direct blood relatives, and note the age and health status, or age at death of each immediate relative. For example, father, deceased, age 67, CVA. Mother, A&W, age 64.

Social History

This portion of the history allows you to learn more about a patient's private lifestyle practices and activities of daily living, while identifying potential risk factors. It also provides an opportunity to initiate patient education and promote positive lifestyle changes. Many of the topics covered are of a sensitive nature so you may want to preface this discussion by reassuring your patient that these questions are part of a routine history and they are asked of all patients.

Tobacco Use

Documented as pack years: number of packs smoked daily × years smoked. If a patient reports they were a former smoker, document their pack years and quit date.

Alcohol

Document consumption quantity and frequency. For example, Do you consume any alcohol, and, if so, how often? Determine the type: beer, liquor, or wine; the volume consumed; and the frequency. If a red flag is raised that the patient may have alcohol dependence or addiction, continue the conversation by asking the CAGE questionnaire.[2]

- Have you ever felt you needed to **C**ut down on your drinking?
- Have people **A**nnoyed you by criticizing your drinking?
- Have you ever felt **G**uilty about your drinking?
- Have you ever felt you needed a drink first thing in the morning (**E**ye-opener) to steady your nerves or to get rid of a hangover?

If a patient answers yes to two or more questions, this is considered clinically significant, and further evaluation and treatment regarding alcohol abuse is recommended.

Illicit Drug Use

Document specific drug, quantity, and frequency. For example, Do you ever use drugs that are not prescribed to you? This includes marijuana, cocaine, heroin, etc. If so, determine the frequency and volume of consumption.

Occupation

Is the patient currently employed? If employed, is it on a full-time, part-time, or per diem basis. Does their profession in any way influence why they are present for this visit? If unemployed, for what length of time have they been out of work?

Functional Status and Independence

Do they live alone, with family, friends, or in an assisted living facility? Can they prepare their own meals and bathe independently? Are there stairs in their home, and can they be navigated safely? Do they drive a motor vehicle? Do they feel safe at home? If pertinent, you may also discuss: diet, sleep, religion, sexual status and activity, education, and military involvement.

Current Medications

All current prescribed and over-the-counter medications or supplements should be listed in the patient record. Complete documentation includes: name of the medication, dosage, route and frequency of administration, and length of time patient has been taking the medication. For example, Metformin 500 mg, 1 tablet po, once daily, ×3 years.

Some other medications that are relevant to orthopaedics that can affect bone and soft-tissue health include: steroids, bisphosphonates, calcitonin, estrogen, parathyroid hormone, chemotherapy, nonsteroidal anti-inflammatories, proton pump inhibitors, and fluoroquinolones. It is important to document if your patient has taken any of these medications in the past, for what length of time, and when the medication was discontinued. Chapter 5 will further review these medications and why they are important to each specific class of orthopaedic patient.

Allergies

All food and drug allergies as well as reaction type and severity of the reaction must be documented. Many patients often, consider mild side effects of medications to be an allergy. For example, nausea is a common side effect many patients experience to narcotic medications. It is important to note such effects so you can determine the optimal medication to prescribe for your patient, but do understand this is not a true allergy. Be sure to delineate true allergies from adverse reactions. In addition, ask patients if they have experienced any metal sensitivity. This is commonly recognized when patients have a reaction to costume jewelry. Because many orthopaedic patients may be operative candidates acutely or in the future, this information is important to help tailor which implants are selected for them. Often patients will indicate that they are uncertain of any sensitivity. You can further explore this possibility by asking if they have dental implants or a pacemaker or defibrillator.

III. PHYSICAL EXAMINATION

The physical examination for an acute musculoskeletal trauma patient will differ from that of a new patient seen in the outpatient office setting. Below is an example of a comprehensive outpatient or clinic physical examination. First remember to wash your hands and to follow necessary precautions for the given patient. Most patients will require standard gloves only. If you expect possible soiling, gowning is also advised. For open wounds or examinations requiring a procedure, sterile gloves are advised. Other precautions include: contact, enteric, droplet, airborne, and airborne respirator for which you must follow specific protocol. Before completing each portion of the examination, explain to the patient what you are going to do. If the patient is not able to be evaluated in their clothing, provide gown or loose shorts to allow necessary skin exposure.

General Survey

This portion of the examination comments on the overall appearance and well-being of the patient. Is the patient alert and oriented? Note their level of distress: no acute distress, mild, moderate, severe. Signs of distress include: crying, grimacing, groaning, and difficulty breathing. Behavior: are they anxious, agitated, cooperative, uncooperative, or withdrawn? Hydration status: well hydrated, dehydrated? Ambulation status: Normal gait, abnormal gait, use of assertive devices, wheelchair bound, bed bound? Do they appear well nourished, malnourished, or obese? Are they well kept or disheveled in appearance? Does their breath smell of: acetone, alcohol, smoke?

Vital Signs

Always document temperature (97°F to 100.4°F), pulse (60 and 100 beats/min), blood pressure (100/60 to 140/90), respiratory rate (12 and 20 respirations/min), and blood oxygen saturation (>93%). These measurements may identify an acute medical problem or evaluate a chronic medical condition. Often vital signs can be overlooked in an outpatient setting, but remember, vital signs are *always* vital. The patient's height and weight should also be measured and BMI calculated. Pre-hypertension is a systolic blood pressure 120 to 140 mm Hg or diastolic blood pressure 80 to 90 mm Hg, whereas hypertension is a systolic blood pressure >140 mm Hg or diastolic blood pressure >90 mm Hg.

Ophthalmologic

Note presence of: pupils equal, round, reactive to light and accommodative, Extraoccular muscles intact, and normal conjunctiva.

Head, Ears, Nose, Throat

Is the patient normocephalic, atraumatic? Does the patient have normal hearing? Nasal discharge? Evaluate the oral mucosa: dry, erythematous? Note dentition.

Neck

Is the neck supple? Nontender? Is the trachea midline? Note the presence of lymphadenopathy and thyromegaly. Scars present? Assess active range of motion (Table 4-1).

TABLE 4-1	Full Active Range of Motion of the Neck
Motion	**Typical Range (degrees)**
Flexion	70–90
Extension	60–70
Lateral bending	30–40
Rotation	80–90

Respiratory System
Observation and Inspection
Are their breaths regular and deep? Does their breathing pattern appear labored, distressed, or involve accessory muscles of breathing, that is, scalene, sternocleidomastoid muscles, or trapezium? Are their lips pursed? Evaluate the color of lips and nail beds. Observe their posture. What is their ability to speak? If the patient is unable to speak in complete sentences, count how many words they can speak before taking a breath. Are there any audible noises that do not require use of the stethoscope, that is, wheezing or gurgling?

Evaluate for Chest and Spinal Deformities
Deformities may impair a patient's normal breathing ability. Look for barrel chest (increased AP diameter, associated with emphysema and hyperinflation), pectus excavatum (posterior displacement of the inferior sternum), kyphosis (excessive convexity of the cervical, thoracic, or sacral spine), lordosis (increased concavity of the cervical or lumbar spine), and scoliosis (sideways curvature of the spine).

Palpation of the Chest
Palpation will aid in evaluating chest excursion and to allow you to perform tactile fremitus which may identify lung consolidations or pleural fluid.

Percussion
Striking a surface that covers an air-filled structure (healthy lung) produces a resonant tone vs. displaced tissue full of fluid (pleural effusion) produces a dull tone vs. infiltrated space (pneumonia) which produces a deadened tone.

Auscultation
Remind yourself of lung lobe anatomy. With the patient sitting upright, instruct them to take slow deep breaths through their mouth while auscultating posteriorly then anteriorly for clear lungs (vesicular breath sounds), wheezes (high-pitch whistling sound most pronounced during expiration because of narrowed airways),

rales (scratchy crackling sound most commonly associated with fluid accumulation), or rhonchi (continuous low-pitched rattling sound common with obstruction and secretions). Patients with large breasts may be asked to lay down allowing their breasts to fall to the side improving ability to auscultate the lungs.

Cardiovascular

Observation and Inspection

Evaluate for jugular venous distention which, if present, indicates an increase in central venous pressure and comments on the patient's intravascular volume status and overall cardiac function. Remember the internal jugular vein is located between the two heads of the sternocleidomastoid muscle (SCM) and anterior to the ear. Have you patient turn their head to the left and apply resistance to define the SCM.

Palpation

Determine the point of maximum impulse.

Auscultation

With the diaphragm of your stethoscope, auscultate for S1 and S2. Volume: how loud is the sound? The majority of murmurs are evaluated as 1 to 3/6. Are there additional heart sounds (S3, S4) described as a gallop? In a patient >30 years old, this often indicates pathology.

During the cardiovascular examination, you may also want to evaluate the distal extremities for cardiac dysfunction and peripheral vascular disease or you may save this portion of the examination for the musculoskeletal examination. A brief examination may begin with evaluating for peripheral edema (Table 4-2).

Next evaluate distal pulses to determine the presence of arterial vascular disease (Table 4-3). This includes the dorsalis pedis and the posterior tibial arteries. The dorsalis pedis terminates at the proximal aspect of the first intermetatarsal space. It can be palpated just lateral to the extension hallucis longus tendon just distal to the navicular bone (Figure 4-1). The posterior tibial artery is just posterior to the medial malleolus.

TABLE 4-2	Subjective Edema Grading System
1+	2 mm depression, rebounds immediately, no visible distortion
2+	2–4 mm deep pit, a few seconds to rebound
3+	6 mm deep pit, 10–12 seconds to rebound, extremity appears full and swollen
4+	8 mm, very deep pit, >20 seconds to rebound, extremity is grossly distorted

TABLE 4-3	Subjective Distal Pulse Grading System
0	Not palpable, absent
1	Palpable, thready/weak
2	Normal, easily identified
3	Increased pulse, moderate pressure for obliteration
4	Bounding, cannot obliterate

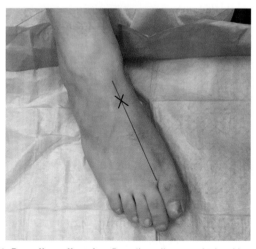

Figure 4-1 **Dorsalis pedis pulse.** Dorsalis pedis artery depicted in red and location of pulse palpation depicted by X.

Lastly, evaluate capillary refill. Press on the nail of the great toe or fingers until blanching occurs. Then, release and measure time for blood inflow to the distal aspect of the lower extremity. Within normal limits: immediate to 2 seconds. Greater than 2 seconds is abnormal and indicates arterial insufficiency or hypovolemia.

Gastrointestinal

Inspect for surgical scars, feeding tubes, and ostomies. Palpate the abdomen and note if it is soft, nontender, and nondistended. Evaluate for organomegaly. Auscultate in all four quadrants for normal bowel sound.

Musculoskeletal Examination

Begin all examinations with inspection for skin changes, edema, erythema, ecchymosis, gross deformity, symmetry compared to the contralateral extremity, muscle atrophy, joint contracture, scars, and position extremity is held in. Muscle strength is graded in the following manner:

- 0/5: no contraction
- 1/5: muscle flicker, but no movement
- 2/5: movement possible, but not against gravity (test the joint in its horizontal plane)
- 3/5: movement possible against gravity, but not against examiner's resistance
- 4/5: movement possible against some resistance by the examiner
- 5/5: normal strength

Upper Extremity Examination

Shoulder and Upper Arm Examination

The glenohumeral joint is the most mobile joint in the body and the arms' connection to the axial skeleton (Figure 4-2). Because the shoulder has a significant amount of multidirectional range of motion, there is great potential for joint instability. Following inspection, continue your examination with palpation of the

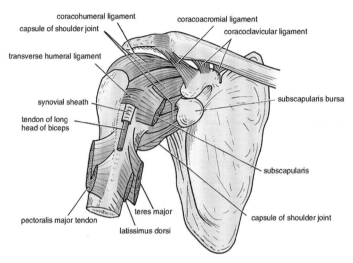

Figure 4-2 Anterior shoulder anatomy. (From Snell RS. *Clinical Anatomy by Regions.* Philadelphia, PA: Wolters Kluwer; 2011.)

bony structures: the sternoclavicular joint, the clavicle, the acromioclavicular (AC) joint, the coracoid process, the borders of the scapula, and the greater and lesser tuberosities of the humerus. Next, palpate the soft-tissue landmarks including: the trapezius, deltoid, infraspinatus, supraspinatus, and teres minor muscles, the subacromial bursa, the supraclavicular fossa, the biceps tendon, and other associated muscles and tendons. Make note of pain, muscle wasting/atrophy, increased warmth, or crepitus.

Next, assess the active range of motion of the shoulder (Table 4-4). The patient may be seated or standing for this examination. If there is no known injury to the shoulders, bilateral examinations may be conducted simultaneously. If the patient is unable to perform AROM of the shoulder joint, a passive range of motion examination may be completed. In some situations, both evaluations are valuable. Pain with AROM but not PROM may indicate muscle or tendon pathology because these structures are not activated during PROM. Note if limitations are due to pain, weakness, or fatigue and how

TABLE 4-4 Shoulder Range of Motion Values		
Motion	**Typical Range**	**Special Instruction**
Forward flexion	0–180 degrees	Perform with elbows in extension
Extension	0–60 degrees	Perform with elbows in extension
Abduction	0–180 degrees	
Cross body adduction	0–45 degrees	
Internal rotation	0–90 degrees	Perform with elbows flexed to 90 degrees and forearm in neutral
External rotation	0–90 degrees	Perform with elbows flexed to 90 degrees and forearm in neutral
Abduction and external rotation	In relation to the cervical spine ~C7	
Adduction and internal rotation	Lower border of the scapula or in relation to the thoracic spine ~T7	

results compare to the contralateral joint. *Remember*, all range of motion measurements should be assessed with a goniometer for precise and reproducible measurements. Lastly, evaluate and grade the strength of the following muscles:

- Deltoid: shoulder abduction
- Subscapularis: test internal rotation, may also evaluate with Lift-off test, see later
- Supraspinatus: test abduction, may also evaluate with Empty Can test, see later
- Teres minor and infraspinatus: test external rotation

Special Tests and Clinical Considerations for the Shoulder

Remember, none of the following tests are 100% sensitive or specific for any particular injury or condition.

Lift-off test (Figure 4-3): Subscapularis muscle and tendon:

Maneuver: Have the patient adduct and internally rotate their arm behind their back with their palm facing away from the back. Instruct them to lift their hand off their lower back.

Positive Examination: Inability to lift the dorsum of hand off the back may be suggestive of complete tear of subscapularis tendon or muscle. Incomplete tear may present as limited lift or pain with lift.

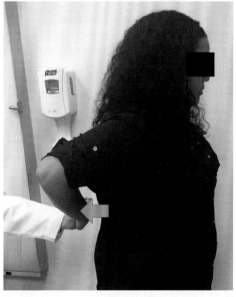

Figure 4-3 Lift-off test. Instruct patient to adduct and internally rotate arm. Then instruct patient to lift hand off lower back in resistance to practitioner. Weakness or inability to lift suggestive of subscapularis tendon or muscle pathology.

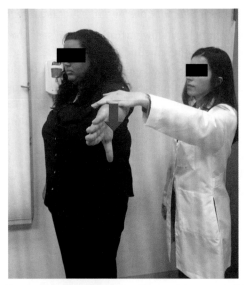

Figure 4-4 **Empty can test.** Instruct the patient to abduct arm to 90 degrees and adduct forward to 30 degrees with the thumbs pointing down toward the floor. Instruct the patient to maintain this position while practitioner applies downward resistance to the patient's forearm. Decreased strength or pain may be suggestive of supraspinatus tendon or muscle pathology.

Empty can test (Figure 4-4): Supraspinatus muscle and tendon:

   Maneuver: Instruct the patient to abduct to 90 degrees and adduct forward to 30 degrees with the thumbs pointing down toward the floor (appears as if pouring out a can). Instruct the patient to maintain this position while the examiner applies downward resistance to the patient's forearms.

   Positive Findings: Decreased strength or pain which may be suggestive of tendon or muscle tear.

External rotators:

   Maneuver: Perform with elbows flexed to 90 degrees and forearm in neutral. Place your hands on the outside of their forearms and instruct the patient to eternally rotate against your resistance.

Positive Examination: Decreased strength or pain may be suggestive of tendon or muscle tear. Significant weakness of the infraspinatus may indicate suprascapular nerve palsy or denervation.

Neer's impingement test (Figure 4-5)*:*

Maneuver: Stabilize the scapula with one hand while grasping the ipsilateral forearm. The arm should be internally rotated with thumb posting down. Passively forward flex the arm to above the head.

Positive Findings: Pain in the anterior shoulder is suggestive of impingement, tendonitis, or bursitis.

Hawkin's impingement test (Figure 4-6):

Maneuver: Instruct the patient to forward flex their arm to 90 degrees and their elbow to 90 degrees. Place one hand on top of the shoulder for stabilization and to prevent elevation while internally rotating the arm at the forearm.

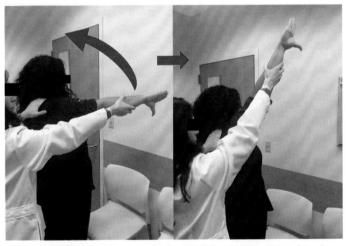

Figure 4-5 Neer's test. Practitioner should stabilize ipsilateral scapula and passively forward flex patient's internally rotated arm with downward pointing thumb. Anterior shoulder pain suggestive of impingement.

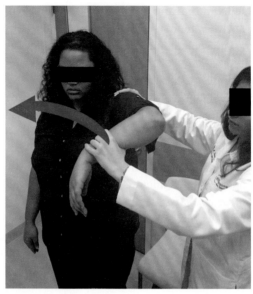

Figure 4-6 Hawkin's test. Instruct the patient to forward flex their arm to 90 degrees and their elbow to 90 degrees. Practitioner should stabilize ipsilateral shoulder while internally rotating the forearm. Anterior shoulder pain suggestive of impingement.

Positive Findings: Pain in the anterior shoulder is suggestive of impingement, tendonitis, or bursitis.

AC joint testing:

Maneuver: Identify the AC joint by palpating laterally along the clavicle until it articulates with the acromion. Gently push on the AC joint, noting if pain is reproducible. Another test is the cross arm adduction test (Figure 4-7).

Maneuver: Instruct the patient to adduct their arm across their chest stressing the AC joint.

Positive Findings: Reproducible pain may be suggestive of arthritis. In the setting of AC separation, the area may appear swollen and deformed when compared with the contralateral joint.

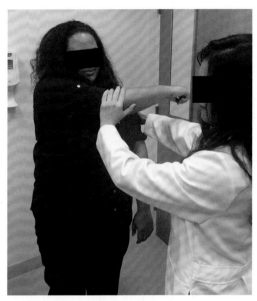

Figure 4-7 **Cross arm test.** Instruct the patient to adduct their arm across their chest stressing the AC joint. Reproducible pain may be suggestive of arthritis.

The apprehension test (Figure 4-8):

Maneuver: Instruct the patient to lie on their back with their arm off the examination table. Hold their elbow flexed at 90 degrees and abduct their shoulder to 90 degrees. While externally rotating their arm, gently push anteriorly on the head of the humerus with your other hand. Then, begin to relocate the humeral head.

Positive Findings: The patient becoming apprehensive, complains of pain, or you feel the humeral head is about to pop out of the glenoid, is suggestive of instability.

Biceps tendonitis: Remember: the biceps muscle functions to supinate and flex the forearm while assisting with forward flexion of the shoulder.

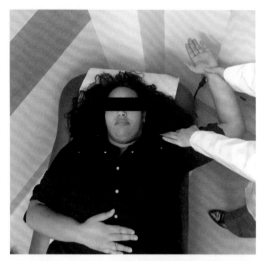

Figure 4-8 **Apprehension test.** Instruct the patient to lie on their back with their arm off the examination table. Hold their elbow flexed at 90 degrees and abduct their shoulder to 90 degrees. While externally rotating their arm, gently push anteriorly on the head of the humerus with your other hand and locate the humeral head. Patient apprehensiveness or pain suggestive of glenohumeral instability.

Maneuver: First, palpate the biceps tendon in the bicipital groove (between the greater and lesser tubercles of the humeral head). If having difficulty locating the tendon, instruct the patient to flex and supinate their forearm while you palpate. Yergason's test: Instruct the patient to flex their elbow to 90 degrees and maintain their shoulder adducted against their body. Grasp the patient's hand and instruct them to supinate their forearm while you provide resistance.

Positive Findings: Pain upon palpation or with Yergason's test may be suggestive of tendonitis.

Speed's test (Figure 4-9):

Maneuver: Instruct the patient to flex their elbow to 30 degrees and supinate their forearm. Then, instruct the patient to further forward flex their shoulder while you provide resistance.

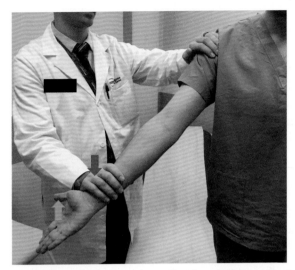

Figure 4-9 **Speed's test.** Instruct patient to flex elbow to 30 degrees and supinate their forearm. Then, instruct patient to flex shoulder against practitioner resistance. Anterior shoulder pain suggestive of biceps tendon pathology.

Positive Findings: Pain in the anterior shoulder with resisted flexion is suggestive of biceps tendonitis.

Biceps tendon rupture: Owing to acute trauma or chronic tendonitis or trauma. On examination, there may be a palpable defect, and the biceps muscle will appear retracted and balled up, referred to as a "Popeye deformity" (Figure 4-10). Examination may also be positive for ecchymosis and edema on the anterior elbow. There will be loss of function most significantly manifested as weakened forearm supination, but also as weakened elbow flexion and forward flexion of the shoulder.

The Elbow and Forearm Examination

Begin with inspection and palpation of the bony structures of the elbow, a hinge-type joint (Figure 4-11). Palpate the medial and lateral epicondyles as well as the olecranon. Then assess active and passive ranges of motion (Table 4-5). Next, evaluate muscle strength. Muscles to evaluate:

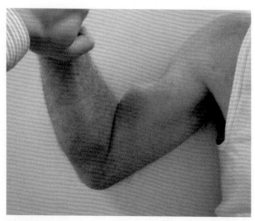

Figure 4-10 Popeye deformity. Popeye deformity demonstrating biceps retraction following biceps tendon rupture.

- Biceps brachii, brachialis: test elbow flexion with hand supinated
- Brachioradialis: test elbow flexion with forearm in natural and thumb pointing up
- Triceps brachii: test elbow extension
- Pronator quadratus, pronator teres, and brachioradialis: test forearm pronation
- Biceps brachii, supinator, and brachioradialis: test forearm supination

Special Tests and Clinical Considerations for the Elbow

Evaluation of lateral epicondylitis (*tennis elbow*) (Figure 4-12):
Remember, the wrist extensors and supinator insert on the lateral epicondyle of the humerus.

Maneuver: First, palpate the lateral epicondyle. Then, instruct the patient to extend their wrist against your resistance.

Positive Findings: Reproducibility of pain with palpation or resistive movement in the absence of erythema or signs of acute infection is suggestive of lateral epicondylitis.

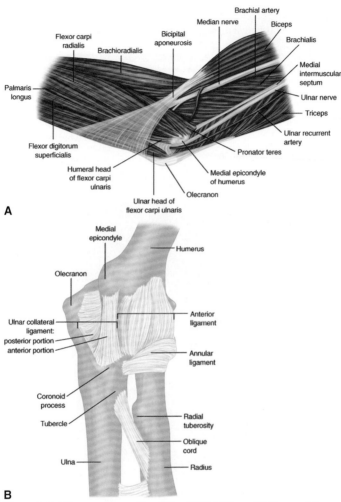

Figure 4-11 Elbow anatomy. (From Wiesel SW, Williams GR, Ramsey ML, Wiesel BB. *Operative Techniques in Shoulder and Elbow Surgery*. 2nd ed. Philadelphia, PA: Wolters Kluwer; 2011.)

Evaluation of medial epicondylitis (*Golfer's elbow*): Wrist flexors and forearm pronators insert on the medial epicondyle.

Maneuver: First, palpate the medial epicondyle. Then, instruct the patient to flex their wrist against your resistance.

TABLE 4-5	Full Active Range of Motion of the Elbow	
Motion	**Typical Range (degrees)**	**Special Instruction**
Flexion	~150	
Extension	0	
Supination	Neutral-90	Maintain arm adducted against body when assessing
Pronation	Neutral-90	Maintain arm adducted against body when assessing

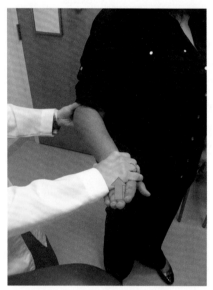

Figure 4-12 Tennis elbow test (Cozen's test). While practitioner palpates patient's lateral epicondyle, instruct patient to extend their wrist against practitioner's resistance. Pain with palpation or resistance suggestive of lateral epicondylitis. Blue arrow is direction of patients resisted motion.

Positive Findings: Reproducibility of pain with palpation or resistive movement in the absence of erythema or signs of acute infection is suggestive of medial epicondylitis.

Ulnar nerve entrapment: At the elbow, the ulnar nerve traverses the groove between the medial epicondyle and olecranon process known as the cubital tunnel. When entrapped, patients report neuropathic pain, that is, pins and needles, electric shock, or weakness in the ulnar nerve distribution. First, assess for normal motor strength: evaluate wrist flexion, finger flexion, and finger adduction/abduction. Next, evaluate for normal sensation utilizing two-point discrimination in the pinky and medial half of the ring finger. Last, perform the ulnar Tinel test (Figure 4-13).

Maneuver: With the elbow slightly flexed at 15 to 20 degrees, tap over the ulnar nerve at the location of the cubital tunnel.

Positive Findings: Tinel's sign: reproducible pain with tapping.

Olecranon bursitis (Figure 4-14): Olecranon bursitis can present as infectious or noninfectious bursitis. Noninfectious bursitis: Often due to trauma, prolonged pressure, ie, persistent leaning on elbow, or excess fluid production within the bursa.

Positive Findings: Swelling at olecranon in the absence of pain, erythema, or warmth with full active painless range of motion.

Infectious bursitis: May result due to cut, abrasion, or insect bite of overlying skin, or other inflammatory processes, ie, rheumatoid arthritis, gout.

Positive Findings: Swelling at olecranon with associated erythema, warmth, and pain on palpation of the bursa. Elbow range of motion is not usually affected.

Evaluation of the lateral collateral ligament, radial collateral ligament:

Maneuver: Instruct the patient to flex their elbow to 20 to 30 degrees with their forearm in neutral position. With the patient's arm stabilized at the medial distal humerus, apply a varus (adduction) force to the distal forearm.

Positive Findings: Pain or excessive gapping compared to contralateral joint may be suggestive of LCL sprain or tear.

Evaluation of the medial collateral ligament (MCL), ulnar collateral ligament:

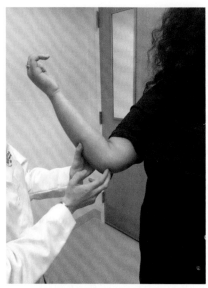

Figure 4-13 Ulnar Tinel sign. Practitioner to gently tap over ulnar nerve traversing the cubital tunnel. Reproducible pain, numbness, or tingling in the median nerve distribution suggestive of ulnar nerve entrapment.

Maneuver: Instruct the patient to flex their elbow to 20 to 30 degrees with their forearm in neutral position. With the patient's arm stabilized at the lateral distal humerus, apply a valgus (abduction) force to the distal forearm.

Positive Findings: Pain or excessive gapping compared to contralateral joint may be suggestive of MCL sprain or tear.

The Wrist and Hand Examination

Begin with inspection and palpation of the bony structures of the wrist and hand. Palpate the distal radius and ulna, radial and ulnar styloids, carpal bones, metacarpophalangeal joints, proximal interphalangeal joints, distal interphalangeal joints, the thumb interphalangeal joint, and the anatomical snuff box (Figure 4-15). Note the presence of Heberden's or Bouchard's nodes, contractures, and thenar, hypothenar, or interossei atrophy. Then, assess active and

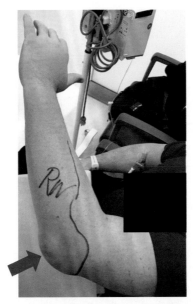

Figure 4-14 Clinical elbow bursitis. Note palpable swelling over olecranon. May be associated with tenderness to palpation. Red arrow points to fluctuant area.

passive ranges of motion (Table 4-6). Be sure to use a finger goniometer for CMC, MCP, PIP, DIP, and IP joints for increased precision in measurement. Next, evaluate muscle strength. Muscles to evaluate:

- Extensor carpi radialis longus: wrist extension
- Flexor carpi radialis and palmaris longus: wrist flexion
- Supinator: wrist supination
- Pronator teres and pronator quadratus: wrist pronation
- Flexor digitorum superficialis: MCP and PIP finger flexion
- Flexor digitorum profundus: DIP flexion
- Extensor digitorum: MCP and IP extension
- Extensor pollicis longus: thumb extension
- Abductor pollicis brevis (APB): thumb abduction
- Flexor pollicis longus: thumb IP flexion
- Dorsal interossei: finger abduction
- Palmar interossei: finger adduction

Figure 4-15 **Hand and wrist anatomy.** (From Tank PW, Gest TR. *Atlas of Anatomy.* Baltimore, MD: Lippincott Williams & Wilkins; 2008.)

Median nerve

Ulnar artery and nerve

Deep palmar branch of ulnar artery

Deep branch of ulnar nerve

Abductor digiti minimi muscle

Superficial branch of ulnar nerve

Flexor digiti minimi brevis muscle

Hypothenar fascia (cut)

Common palmar digital arteries and nerves

Superficial palmar arch

Palmar aponeurosis (reflected)

Proper palmar digital nerves and arteries

Radial artery

Superficial palmar branch of radial artery

Flexor retinaculum

Abductor pollicis brevis muscle

Opponens pollicis muscle

Flexor pollicis brevis muscle

1st lumbrical muscle

Thenar fascia (cut)

Adductor pollicis muscle

Fibrous digital sheath

A

90

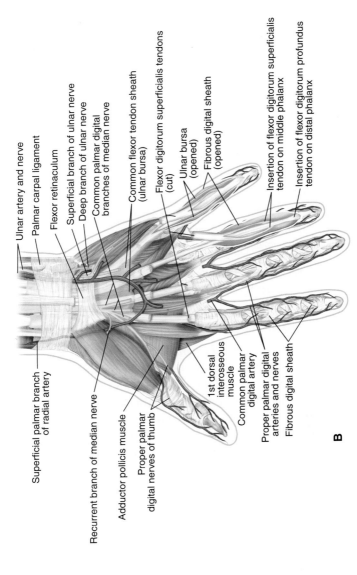

Ulnar artery and nerve

Palmar carpal ligament

Flexor retinaculum

Superficial branch of ulnar nerve

Deep branch of ulnar nerve

Common palmar digital branches of median nerve

Common flexor tendon sheath (ulnar bursa)

Flexor digitorum superficialis tendons (cut)

Ulnar bursa (opened)

Fibrous digital sheath (opened)

Insertion of flexor digitorum superficialis tendon on middle phalanx

Insertion of flexor digitorum profundus tendon on distal phalanx

Superficial palmar branch of radial artery

Recurrent branch of median nerve

Adductor pollicis muscle

Proper palmar digital nerves of thumb

1st dorsal interosseous muscle

Common palmar digital artery

Proper palmar digital arteries and nerves

Fibrous digital sheath

B

Figure 4-15 (continued)

91

TABLE 4-6 Full Active Range of Motion of the Wrist and Hand	
Motion	**Typical Range**
Wrist extension	Neutral-75 degrees
Wrist flexion	Neutral-80 degrees
Radial deviation	Neutral-20 degrees
Ulnar deviation	Neutral-35 degrees
Finger MCP joints	0 degree extension–90 degrees flexion
Finger PIP joints	0 degree extension–100 degrees flexion
Finger DIP joints	0 degree extension–80 degrees flexion
Thumb CMC joint: Palmar adduction/abduction	Contact to 45 degrees
Thumb CMC joint: Radial adduction/abduction	Contact to 60 degrees
Thumb MCP	Hyperextension of 10–55 degrees flexion
Thumb IP	Hyperextension of 15–80 degrees flexion

Special Tests and Clinical Considerations for the Wrist and Hand

Evaluation for carpal tunnel syndrome (median nerve compression):
Inspect the hand for atrophy of the thenar eminence.

Maneuver: Tinel's sign (Figure 4-16): Gently tap over the nerve.

Positive Findings: Reproducible pain or electric shock sensation in the median nerve distribution.

Maneuver: Phalen's sign (Figure 4-17): Instruct the patient to hold their wrist in forced flexion ×1 minute.

Positive Findings: Reproducible pain, numbness, or tingling in the median nerve distribution.

Maneuver: Durkan's carpal tunnel compression test (Figure 4-18): Instruct your patient to rest their hands in a supinated position. Apply direct pressure with your thumb over the carpal tunnel just distal to the wrist crease to increase the pressure for 30 seconds.

Positive Findings: Reproducible pain, numbness, or tingling in the median nerve distribution.

Test the APB muscle for strength (Figure 4-19): Remember: the APB is solely innervated by the median nerve.

Maneuver: Instruct your patient to rest their hand in a supinated position on the examination table and to abduct their thumb up and away from the plane of the palm while you apply resistance.

Positive Findings: <5/5 muscle strength.

Evaluate grip strength with a dynamometer (Figure 4-20): Approximate average grip strength for a healthy male without deficits is about 100 lb of pressure and for a female 60 lb of pressure.

Evaluation for De Quervain's tendonitis: Repetitive motions, specifically adduction and abduction of the thumb, cause inflammation of the extensor pollicis brevis and abductor pollicis longus tendons. Inspection: the thumb usually appears normal. Swelling and tenderness may be present near the radial styloid overlying the EPB

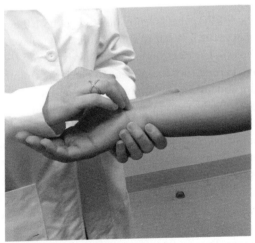

Figure 4-16 Tinel's sign (median nerve). Practitioner to gently tap over median nerve. Reproducible pain, numbness, or tingling in the median nerve distribution suggestive of carpal tunnel syndrome.

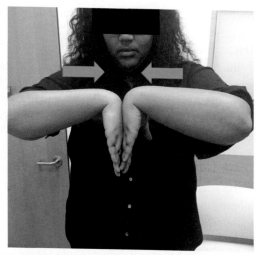

Figure 4-17 Phalen's test. Instruct patient to hold both their wrists in forced flexion against each other. Reproducible pain, numbness, or tingling in the median nerve distribution suggestive of carpal tunnel syndrome. Blue arrows point in direction of force.

and APL. Ask the patient to give you a thumbs up. If they complain of pain over the first dorsal compartment, they have a positive Hitchhiker's sign. Next, perform the Finkelstein test (Figure 4-21):

Maneuver: Instruct the patient to place the thumb in their palm and form a fist. Apply gentle ulnar deviation passively stretching the tendons over the radial styloid.

Positive Findings: Reproducible pain.

Evaluation for ganglion cyst (Figure 4-22): Inspect the structure. Upon palpation, there may or may not be associated tenderness. The structure should feel as a fluid-filled, mobile mass that can transilluminate. Some ganglions are located intimately to either the radial or ulnar arteries. Perform the Allen test to evaluate hand perfusion (Figure 4-23).

Maneuver: The patient is instructed to clench their fist. During this time, the examiner applies pressure over the ulnar and the radial arteries to occlude both of them simultaneously.

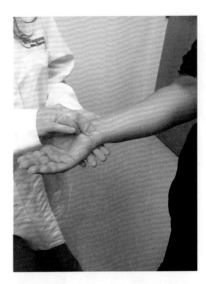

Figure 4-18 Durkan's test. Instruct patient to rest their hands in a supinated position. Apply direct pressure with your thumb over the carpal tunnel just distal to the wrist crease to increase the pressure for 30 seconds. Reproducible pain, numbness, or tingling in the median nerve distribution suggestive of carpal tunnel syndrome.

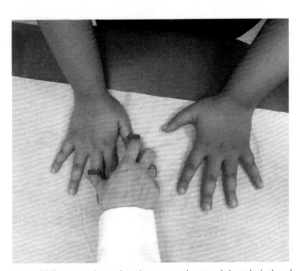

Figure 4-19 APB strength testing. Instruct patient to abduct their thumb against practitioner's resistance. Weakness typically suggestive of median nerve pathology. Red arrow demonstrates examiners resistance force.

Figure 4-20 Hand dynamometer. Evaluation of hand grip strength using hand dynamometer.

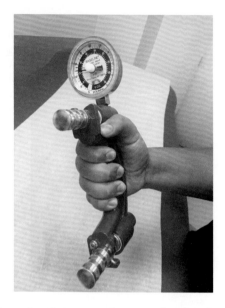

After 30 seconds, the patient is instructed to open their hand. It should appear blanched. Pressure from the ulnar artery is released while radial pressure is maintained. Rubor should return to the hand immediately. Repeat this examination releasing pressure from the radial artery while ulnar pressure is maintained. Document the time for rubor to return.

Positive Findings: If pallor persists for greater than 3 seconds after the patient opens their fingers and arterial pressure is released, this is suggestive of some degree of occlusion of the uncompressed artery.

Evaluating for intersection syndrome: Repetitive motions such as wrist flexion and extension precipitate this syndrome. The patient will often complain of radial wrist and forearm pain approximately 4 cm proximal to Lister's tubercle. Palpate this location for reproducible pain, which may be suggestive of tenosynovitis. This location represents the crossing over of the abductor pollicis longus and extensor pollicis brevis muscle bellies over the second compartment extensor carpi radialis longus and extensor carpi radialis brevis. Also, evaluate the forearm for swelling.

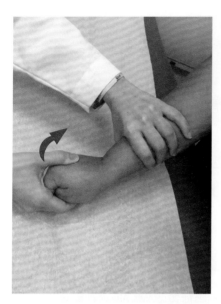

Figure 4-21 Finkelstein's maneuver. Instruct patient to form a fist with their thumb in their palm. Practitioner should ulnar deviate the patient's wrist. Reproducible pain over the radial styloid suggestive of De Quervain's tenosynovitis. Red arrow depicts ulnar directed force at the wrist.

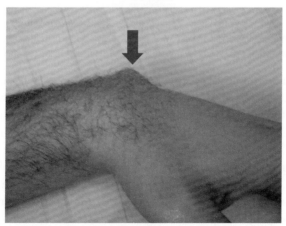

Figure 4-22 Clinical ganglion cyst. Note cystic mass (Red arrow). Mass typically mobile and may be tender to palpation.

Evaluation for wrist stability: Watson's test for scapholunate dysfunction: Instruct the patient to rest their elbow on the examination table with their elbow flexed to about 90 degrees and their forearm in the air.

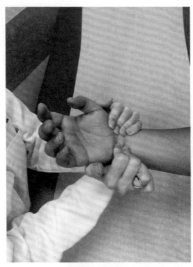

Figure 4-23 **Allen's test.** Instruct the patient to clench their fist and apply pressure over ulnar and radial arteries for 30 seconds. Afterward, instruct patient to open their hand and release pressure from the ulnar artery while radial pressure is maintained and document time for return to rubor. Repeat examination and release radial pressure before ulnar pressure. Persistent pallor >3 seconds after arterial pressure is released suggestive of some occlusion in the uncompressed artery.

Maneuver: Place your thumb over the distal pole of the scaphoid (palmar aspect). Begin with the maximum hand ulnar deviation and slight extension. Apply constant pressure with your thumb and passively move the wrist to a position of radial deviation and slight flexion.

Positive Findings: Reproducible dorsal wrist pain or a clunk may be suggestive of scapholunate ligament tear and instability.

Evaluation for infectious flexor tenosynovitis: The patient may present complaining of pain, swelling, and loss of range of motion in one or several fingers. Evaluate the palmar aspect of the finger for swelling and erythema and position of comfort finger is held in. Palpate for crepitus along the course of the flexor tendon during active and passive flexion of the digit. Next, compare active and passive ranges of motion for discrepancies.

Positive Findings: Fusiform swelling, erythema, semiflexed position, severe pain with passive extension, palpable crepitus, and tenderness along the flexor tendon sheath only.

Evaluation for ECU subluxation: This may be isolated or exist with ECU tendinitis.

Maneuver: Palpate the ECU tendon while instructing the patient to actively rotate their forearm from full supination to pronation with the wrist in a neutral position.

Positive Findings: Subluxation of the ECU on supination with ulnar deviation, audible snap may present. When pronated the ECU relocates into its normal sulcus.

Evaluation for trigger finger (Figure 4-24): Narrowing or inflammation of the tendon sheath, inflammation of the tendon, or nodular

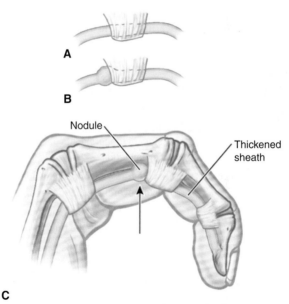

Figure 4-24 Trigger finger. Flexor tendon anatomy and pulley system demonstrating inflammation of the tendon sheath. (From Anderson MK. *Foundations of Athletic Training.* Philadelphia, PA: Wolters Kluwer; 2016.)

formation preventing smooth flexion and extension of the finger. Inspection: the palm and fingers usually appear normal. First, palpate the palm over the A1 pulley. Note tenderness or palpable lump.

Maneuver: Instruct the patient to fully flex the affected finger followed by full extension.

Positive Findings: Impaired movement, pain or active triggering. Grading of trigger finger ranges from 1 to 6 based on severity (Table 4-7).

Evaluation for a mallet finger: The disruption of the terminal extensor tendon distal to DIP joint. Mallet finger injuries may be bony or tendinous. Instruct the patient to actively extend the finger.

Positive Findings: The DIP joint will remain flexed at approximately 45 degrees, lack of active DIP extension.

Evaluation for collateral ligament injuries of the thumb: UCL injuries (Gamekeeper's thumb or Skier's thumb) are significantly more common than RCL injuries. Inspect the thumb for swelling. Then palpate the MCP joint of the thumb for reproducible pain and

TABLE 4-7	Grading of Trigger Finger[3]	
Grade 1	Pretriggering	History of triggering, but not demonstrable on examination
Grade 2	Active	Demonstrable triggering, patient can actively overcome the trigger
Grade 3	Passive	Demonstrable trigger, patient cannot actively overcome the trigger
Grade 3A	Extension	Locked in flexion, needs passive extension to overcome trigger
Grade 3B	Flexion	Locked in extension, needs passive flexion to overcome trigger
Grade 4	Contracture	Demonstrable trigger with flexion contracture of PIP

a possible mass (torn ligament or bony avulsion). Last, stress the joint with a radial deviated motion and compare to the contralateral joint for instability.

Froment's sign (Figure 4-25):

> **Maneuver:** Instruct the patient to grasp a piece of paper between their index finger and thumb (pinch grip). Then, pull on the paper to remove it from the patient's hand. Examine the IP joint while performing.
>
> **Positive Findings:** Flexion of the IP joint may be suggestive of an ulnar nerve weakness.

Wartenberg's sign: Involuntary abduction of the little finger. The presence of this sign is suggestive of weakness of the ulnar innervated intrinsic muscles and unopposed action of the EDQ.

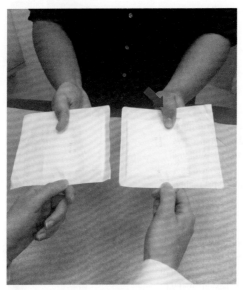

Figure 4-25 Froment's sign. Instruct the patient to grasp a piece of paper between their index finger and thumb (pinch grip). Practitioner is to then pull on the paper and examine the IP joint while doing. Flexion of the IP joint (indicated by red arrow) may be suggestive of an ulnar nerve weakness.

Sensation Examination

Each dermatome must be assessed for thorough evaluation of sensation (Figure 4-26). Note if sensation is intact to light touch in the axillary, musculocutaneous, lateral antebrachial and medial antebrachial cutaneous, median, radial, and ulnar distributions. Two-point discrimination (Figure 4-27) should also be evaluated. Note the maximum distance at which the patient can identify two nearby sharp objects as two truly distinct points, not one.

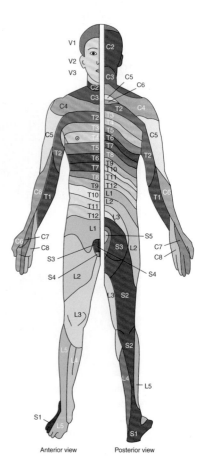

Figure 4-26 **Dermatomes.** Anterior and posterior views of the dermatomes. Although dermatomes are shown as distinct segments, in reality, there is overlap between any two adjacent dermatomes. The sensory innervation of the face does not involve dermatomes but instead is carried by cranial nerve (CN) V; V1 (ophthalmic division), V2 (maxillary division), and V3 (mandibular division). (From Moore KL, Dalley AF, Agur AMR. *Clinically Oriented Anatomy*. 7th ed. Philadelphia, PA: Lippincott Williams & Wilkins; 2014:51.)

Anterior view   Posterior view

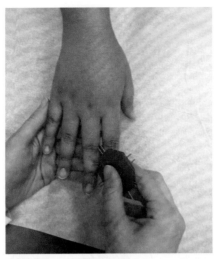

Figure 4-27 Two-point discrimination test. Practitioner should gently roll two-point discriminator wheel on patient's skin. The maximum distance with which patient can identify two distinct points should be noted in assessment of sensation.

Vascular Examination

Be familiar with the vasculature of the upper extremity (Figure 4-28). First, inspect the extremity: Does it appear pink, perfused and feel warm? Or is it cool to the touch, dusky and with pallor? Has a portion of the limb become necrotic? Assess for brachial, radial, and ulnar pulses, and grade accordingly. Partially flexing the patients' wrist may aid in detecting radial and ulnar pulses. To locate the patient brachial pulse, flex their elbow slightly and palpate medial to the biceps tendon in the antecubital crease. If unable to palpate pulses, use a Doppler ultrasonic probe for pulse detection. Also, comment on capillary refill. Remember, a normal examination reveals perfusion in <2 seconds.

Spinal Examination

In order to perform an accurate history and physical examination on a spine patient, it is important to understand the spine and its different segments. The vertebral column refers to the skeletal aspect of the spine that protects the spinal cord and which consists of 7 cervical vertebrae, 12 thoracic vertebrae, 5 lumbar vertebrae,

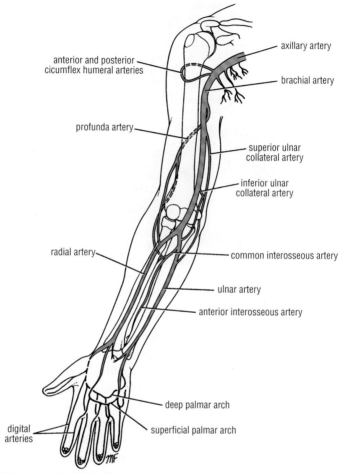

anterior and posterior cicumflex humeral arteries

axillary artery

brachial artery

profunda artery

superior ulnar collateral artery

inferior ulnar collateral artery

radial artery

common interosseous artery

ulnar artery

anterior interosseous artery

deep palmar arch

digital arteries

superficial palmar arch

Figure 4-28 Upper extremity vasculature. Upper extremity arterial blood supply. (From Snell RS. *Clinical Anatomy.* 7th ed. Philadelphia, PA: Lippincott, Williams & Wilkins; 2003.)

the sacrum, and the coccyx. The spinal cord is composed of nerve roots, which exit the spinal cord at each segmental level. The cervical spine is composed of 8 nerve roots, the thoracic spine of 12 nerve roots, the lumbar spine of 5 nerve roots, and the sacrum of 5 nerve roots (Figure 4-29). The C5–T1 nerves innervate the upper

Figure 4-29 Spinal cord nerve roots. There are 8 nerve roots exiting the cervical spine, 12 exiting the thoracic spine, 5 exiting the lumbar spine, and 5 exiting the sacrum (LifeART image copyright (c) 2017. Lippincott Williams & Wilkins. All rights reserved.)

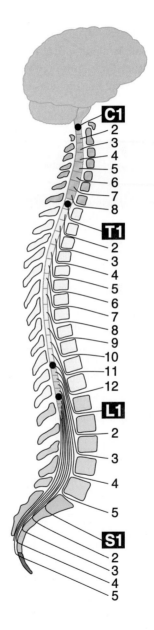

extremities (Table 4-8), and the L1–S4 nerve roots innervate the lower extremities along with bowel and bladder function (Table 4-9).

The history for a spine patient is very similar to a general orthopaedic visit, but includes several questions specific to the

TABLE
4-8

Cervical Spine Motor/Sensory Testing[4]

Motion	Muscle	Innervation	
Shoulder abduction	Deltoid	Axillary nerve	C5
Shoulder internal rotation	Subscapularis	Subscapular nerve	C5
Shoulder external rotation	Infraspinatus	Subscapular nerve	C5
Elbow flexion	Biceps and brachial	Musculocutaneous nerve	C5
Elbow flexion	Brachioradialis	Radial nerve	C6
Elbow extension	Triceps	Radial nerve	C7
Wrist extension	ECRL	Radial nerve	C6
Wrist supination	Supinator	Radial nerve—deep branch	C6
Wrist flexion	FCR and PL	Median nerve	C7
Wrist pronation	PT and PQ	Median nerve	C7
MPC and PIP finger flexion	FDS	Median nerve	C8
DIP flexion	FDP	Ulnar nerve	C8
MCP and IP extension	Extensor digitorum	Radial nerve—PIN	C7, C8
Thumb extension	EPL	Radial nerve—PIN	C7, C8
Thumb abduction	APB	Median nerve—recurrent branch	C8, T1

TABLE 4-8

Cervical Spine Motor/Sensory Testing[4] (continued)

Motion	Muscle	Innervation	
Thumb IP flexion	FPL	Median nerve—anterior interosseous	C7, C8, T1
Thumb adduction (IP joint)	Adductor pollicis	Ulnar nerve—deep branch	C8, T1
Finger adduction	Palmar interossei	Ulnar nerve—deep branch	C8, T1
Finger abduction	Dorsal interossei	Ulnar nerve—deep palmar branch	C8, T1

TABLE 4-9

Lumbar Motor/Sensory Testing[5]

Innervation	Primary Motion	Primary Muscles	Sensation	Reflex
L1			Iliac crest, groin	Cremasteric
L2, L3	Hip flexion	Iliopsoas (lumbar plexus, femoral nerve)	Anterior and inner thigh	None
	Hip adduction	Hip adductors (obturator nerve)		
L4	Knee extension (also L3)	Quadriceps (femoral nerve)	Lateral thigh, anterior knee, and medial leg	Patellar

(continued)

TABLE 4-9

Lumbar Motor/Sensory Testing[5] (*continued*)

Innervation	Primary Motion	Primary Muscles	Sensation	Reflex
L5	Ankle dorsiflexion (also L4)	Tibialis anterior (deep perineal nerve)	Lateral leg and dorsal foot	None
	Foot inversion	Tibialis posterior (tibial nerve)		
	Toe dorsiflexion	EHL, EDL (DPN)		
	Hip extension	Hamstrings (tibial nerve) and gluteus maximus (inferior gluteal nerve)		
	Hip abduction	Gluteus media (superior gluten nerve)		
S1	Foot plantar flexion Foot eversion	Gastroc-soleus (tibial nerve) Peroneals (SPN)	Posterior leg	Achilles
S2	Toe plantar flexion	FHL, FDL (tibial nerve)	Plantar foot	None
S3, S4	Bowel and bladder function	Bladder	Perianal	

spine. In addition to understanding the chief complaint, it is crucial to find out where exactly the patient's pain is because this can correlate to the nerve level being affected. Ask the patient to trace with their finger exactly where the pain is located or travels. Because nerve compression can cause radicular symptoms, determine if the patient is having arm/leg pain and if so, which arm or leg. Also, document associated neurologic symptoms including numbness, tingling, weakness, saddle anesthesia, and urinary or bowel incontinence.

The physical examination for the spine patient varies based on the patient's chief complaint. Begin the physical examination with inspection of the patient. It is important to take note of symmetry, alignment in sagittal and coronal planes, prior surgical scars, skin defects, and muscle atrophy. Next palpate for local tenderness throughout the spinal axis. Be sure to palpate along the spinous processes and note any step-offs or deformities. Following palpation, evaluate the patient's range of motion. Document range of motion with flexion, extension, lateral bend, and rotation (Table 4-10). Motor testing is crucial in the physical examination and should be repeated frequently to assess for any change in strength. Motor power is transported in the spinal cord along the corticospinal tracts. If the nerve root becomes interrupted or damaged, denervation and paralysis can occur along that myotome. Grade key muscles from 0 to 5 based on the

TABLE 4-10 Full Active Range of Motion of the Spine	
Motion	**Typical Range (degrees)**
Flexion	50
Extension	60
Lateral bend	45
Rotation	80

ASIA grading system. It is important to test muscles from each nerve root group. Based on the ASIA muscle grading system, the following numbers correlate with the patient's motor function on examination: 0 (paralysis), 1 (palpable or visible contraction), 2 (active movement with gravity fully eliminated), 3 (active movement against gravity), 4 (active movement with some resistance), and 5 (active movement with normal resistance).

Immediately following the motor examination is the sensory examination. It is important to evaluate sensation along the dermatomal distributions. Sensation of pain and temperature is transported along the lateral spinothalamic tract. Touch is transported along the ventral spinothalamic tract. Damage to the spinal cord or nerve roots can result in decreased sensation to touch, followed by sensation of pain. The sensory examination is based off of the ASIA sensory grading system: 0 (absent), 1 (impaired), 2 (normal), and NT (not testable). There are two major sensory types in the neurologic examination, which include: pain (prick with sharp object) and light touch (stroke lightly with a finger). There are three minor sensory types, which include: vibration, temperature, and two-point discrimination.

Deep tendon reflexes are another important part of the neurologic examination (Table 4-11). It is important to assess the

TABLE 4-11

Deep Tendon Reflexes and Corresponding Nerve Root

Reflex	Corresponding Nerve Root
Biceps reflex	C5, C6
Brachioradialis	C6
Triceps	C7
Cremasteric	L1
Patellar	L3, L4
Achilles	S1

TABLE 4-12	Reflex Grading System
Grade	**Action**
0	Absent reflex
1	Trace
2	Normal
3	Brisk
4	Unsustained clonus
5	Sustained clonus

reflexes in both extremities for comparison. Just like the motor and sensory examinations, reflexes are based off of a grading system (Table 4-12).

Special Test: Cervical and Lumbar Spine

Spurling's test (Figure 4-30): A provocative test that evaluates for cervical foraminal stenosis.

Maneuver: Rotate the patient's head toward the affected side, extend the neck, and then apply downward pressure on the patient's head.

Positive Findings: Patient complaint of pain radiating down the ipsilateral arm can be suggestive of cervical foraminal stenosis.

Hoffman's test: A test that is sensitive but not specific for cervical myelopathy.

Maneuver: Instruct the patient to relax their hand. Then, while holding the middle phalanx of the third digit, flick the distal phalanx into an extended position.

Positive Findings: Involuntary contraction of the thumb interphalangeal joint.

L'hermitte sign:

Maneuver: Instruct the patient to actively flex their cervical spine. Then extend the cervical spine.

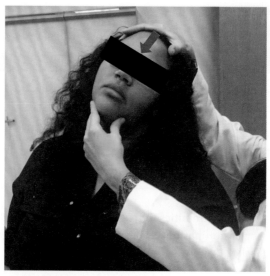

Figure 4-30 **Spurling's test.** Practitioner to rotate the patient's head toward the affected side, extend the neck, and then apply downward pressure on the patient's head (Red arrow). Patient complaints of pain radiating down the ipsilateral arm can be suggestive of cervical foraminal stenosis.

Positive Findings: The patient reports a shocking sensation radiating down the spinal axis into their arms/legs. This finding is suggestive of cervical spinal cord compression and myelopathy.

Straight leg raise (Figure 4-31):

Maneuver: Have the patient lie supine on the examination table. Then instruct them to elevate their leg keeping their knee fully extended. The examiner may passively perform the motion (hip flexion) by cupping the heal and raising.

Positive Findings: If pain or paresthesias are reproducible in the affected leg with 30 to 70 degrees of hip flexion. This test is specific to the lumbar spine and is a tension sign for the L4 and S1 nerve root.

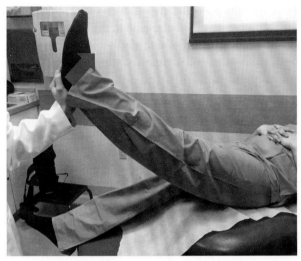

Figure 4-31 **Straight leg raise.** With patient lying supine on examination table practitioner should passively raise patient's fully extended leg by the heel. Reproducible pain, numbness, or tingling when hip is flexed from 30 to 70 degrees suggestive of L5-S1 nerve root pathology. Red arrow depicts force of examiner at the heel.

It is very important to remember when examining a spine patient that details matter. Nerve root compression can affect very specific distributions. With a thorough history and physical examination, you can usually obtain a diagnosis based off of your examination findings. Imaging studies are then important tools to help confirm what you discovered on your examination.

Common Spine Conditions

One of the most common spine condition evaluated and treated is lumbar disc herniation. Disc herniations are more common in men, and usually occur during the fourth and fifth decade of life. About 95% of lumbar disc herniations occur at the L4-L5 or L5-S1 level. Disc herniations generally result from repetitive strain on the outer layer of the disc called the annulus, which then leads to herniation of the center portion of the disc called the nucleus pulposus. Patients generally present with the chief complaint of lumbar pain as well as radicular pain in the buttock and/or legs. Radicular pain is generally made worse with prolonged sitting, coughing, or sneezing and is improved with standing. On physical examination, it is important to test motor strength and sensation of the lower extremities. A straight leg raise is also helpful in diagnosing disc herniations. To definitively diagnose a disc herniation, the gold standard is MRI of the lumbar spine without contrast. First-line treatment for lumbar disc herniations involves physical therapy and anti-inflammatories. About 90% of disc herniations will improve without surgery. Second-line treatment involves selective nerve root corticosteroid injections. If a patient fails nonoperative treatment measures, surgery is considered a third-line treatment to remove the disc herniation.

Lumbar stenosis generally occurs in patients over the age of 50. Stenosis causes a decrease in the central or lateral dimensions of the spinal canal. This narrowing can result from bony structures (osteophytes, uncinate spurs, or spondylolisthesis) or soft-tissue structures (herniated or bulging discs, hypertrophy of ligamentum flavum, or synovial facet cysts). Depending on the severity of the stenosis, patients can present with lumbar back pain, buttock pain, leg pain, claudication, weakness, and bladder disturbances. A thorough physical examination is important to help determine the level at which the stenosis is occurring. Diagnostic imaging plays an important role in obtaining a definitive diagnosis. X-rays of the lumbar spine are helpful to evaluate for bony structure deformities, but an MRI of the lumbar spine without contrast will be the most specific in diagnosing lumbar stenosis and identifying the levels affected. Treatment begins with first-line therapies such as physical therapy and anti-inflammatories. Second-line treatment involves corticosteroid injections. Surgery is a third-line treatment option for patients whose pain persists greater than 3 to 6 months and who have failed nonoperative measures.

Cauda equina syndrome is not only a rare condition of the spine but also a medical emergency. Cauda equina syndrome results from severe compression of the nerve roots. Patients with cauda equina can present with common complaints such as back pain, radicular pain, and paresthesias; most notably patients will complain of bowel and bladder disturbances (incontinence or retention) and saddle anesthesia. It is important to do a rectal examination to document if the patient has normal tone and sensation. With cauda equina syndrome, a patient will have a diminished or absent anal wink test. It is also important to examine the genitalia and test the bulbocavernosus reflex. MRI is the diagnostic test of choice to evaluate for nerve compression. Treatment for cauda equina requires urgent surgical decompression.

The Lower Extremity Examination

The Hip and Upper Leg

As always, begin your examination with inspection. In addition to the standard inspection, you may also evaluate true leg length (measure from the ASIS to the medial malleolus of the ipsilateral leg). If the patient is able, ask them to stand for further inspection of alignment and rotation, then ask the patient to walk 6 to 10 full strides. Assess for gait dysfunction. Remember that a normal gait cycle has two phases, the stance phase and the swing phase. The stance phase begins with the heal strike and ends with the toe off, whereas the swing phase begins with toe off and ends with the heal strike. The gait should appear symmetric, rhythmic, and smooth without apparent discomfort. If the gait does not appear normal, try to discern which phase of the cycle is abnormal, and how the patient is compensating for their pain, weakness, or injury (Table 4-13).

Next, palpate anteriorly. This includes the ASIS, the pubic symphysis, the neurovascular structures (femoral artery, vein, and nerve), and muscles. Laterally palpate the greater trochanteric bursa and the iliac crests. Posteriorly palpate the PSIS, SI joint, ischial tuberosity, and gluteal muscles (Figure 4-32). Most hip joint pathology will not be palpable; however, you may ask the patient to point with one finger to the site of the greatest amount of pain. Next, assess active and passive ranges of motion (Table 4-14) and muscle strength. Muscles to evaluate:

- Iliopsoas (psoas major and iliacus), rectus femoris: hip flexion
- Gluteus maximus: hip extension
- Gluteus medius and minimus: hip abduction
- Adductor brevis, longus and magnus, gracilis: hip adduction

TABLE 4-13

Common Gait Abnormalities and Their Features

Type	Common Characteristics	Cause of Abnormality	Inciting Injuries
Antalgic gait	Shortened stance phase on the affected side	Pain	DJD, subluxation, dislocation, AVN, stress fracture
Trendelenberg gait	When weight is on affected leg (stance phase), contralateral hip drops (hemipelvis tilts down)	Abductor weakness (gluteus medius)	Abductor tear, severe deconditioning, neurologic disorder (superior gluteal nerve)
Abductor lurch (often associated with Trendelenburg gait)	Shortened stance phase while leaning the trunk lurches forward over the affected leg	Effort to compensate	Advanced DJD

TABLE 4-13	Common Gait Abnormalities and Their Features (*continued*)		
Type	**Common Characteristics**	**Cause of Abnormality**	**Inciting Injuries**
Broad based	Irregular steps: uncertain starting and stopping, lateral deviations, unsteady	Cerebellar disease	MS, toxic/metabolic causes, neoplasms, immune mechanisms, trauma
High stepping/ stoppage gait (dorsiflexor)	Difficulty in clear toes doing the swing phase, leg is externally rooted and hip and knee flexed	Loss of proprioception, drop foot	Drop foot
Parkinsonian gait	Short steps, reduced arm swing, stooped posture, anteropulsion/ retropulsion, festination	Bradykinesia	Parkinson disease

- Gluteus medius and minimus, tensor fasciae latae: internal rotation
- Piriformis, gluteus maximus, gemellus superior, quadratus femoris, obturator externus: external rotation

Special Tests for the Sacroiliac Joint

FABER test (*Flexion, ABduction, External Rotation*) (Figure 4-33)

Maneuver: Place the patient's knee in a figure of four position (examining leg ankle on the contralateral knee). Place one

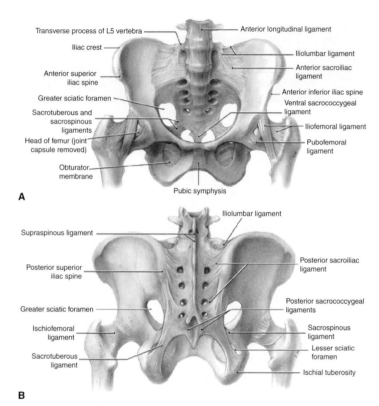

Figure 4-32 **Bony anatomy of the pelvis and hip.** (From Karageanes SJ. *Principles of Manual Sports Medicine.* Philadelphia, PA: Lippincott Williams & Wilkins; 2004.)

hand on the contralateral iliac crest and stabilize the pelvis against the examination table. Apply pressure to relax the knee out by externally rotating the hip.

Positive Findings: Inability to lower the thigh to the table may represent iliopsoas tightness. Reproducible pain by location may be suggestive of:

- SI joint: SI joint dysfunction or sacroiliitis.
- Posterior hip: posterior hip impingement.
- Groin pain: iliopsoas strain or an intra-articular hip condition.

TABLE 4-14	Full Active Range of Motion of the Hip
Motion	**Typical Range (degrees)**
Flexion	0–120
Extension	0–30
Abduction	0–45
Adduction	0–30
Internal rotation	0–45
External rotation	0–45

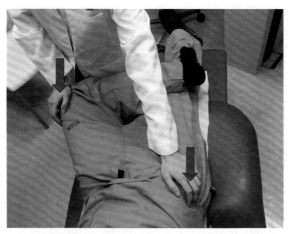

Figure 4-33 FABER (Flexion, ABduction, External Rotation) examination: Instruct patient to lay supine on examination table with ipsilateral knee flexed in figure four position. With one hand stabilizing the contralateral iliac crest (Red arrow to the right), practitioner should apply pressure to the flexed knee resulting in external rotation of the hip. Inability to externally rotate thigh (Red arrow to the left) to table may be suggestive of SI joint pathology, posterior hip impingement, iliopsoas pathology, among others.

Trendelenburg sign: Instruct the patient to stand on one leg (the affected side).

> **Positive Findings:** Dropping of the contralateral PSIS. This may be suggestive of hip abductor and gluteal medius weakening.

Evaluation for trochanteric bursitis: Remember, the trochanteric bursa overlies the greater trochanter of the femur. The patient may complain of lateral or vague hip pain that is worsened by activity. Palpate directly over the bursa for reproducible tenderness.

> **Maneuver:** Instruct the patient to lie on the unaffected side in the lateral decubitus position. Then, ask them to abduct the affected hip while the examiner provides resistance.

> **Positive Findings:** Reproducible pain over the greater trochanter.

Ober's test (Figure 4-34)

> **Maneuver:** Instruct the patient to lie in the lateral decubitus position with the unaffected side against the examination table. Place one hand on the patient's ankle and the other hand over the iliac crest at the lateral hip. Then, passively flex the knee to 90 degrees while extending and abducting the hip. Then, slowly adduct the hip.

> **Positive Findings:** If the patient is unable to undergo passive hip adduction past the midline, it may be suggestive of IT band syndrome or an external snapping hip.

Anterior labral tear testing:

> **Maneuver:** Begin with the hip in a fully flexed, externally rotated, and abducted position and transition to a position of extension, internal rotation, and adduction.

> **Positive Findings:** Reproducible pain, locking, or snapping may be suggestive of an anterior labral tear.

Posterior labral tear testing:

> **Maneuver:** Begin with the hip in a flexed, adducted, and internally rotated position and transition to a position of abduction, external rotation, and extension.

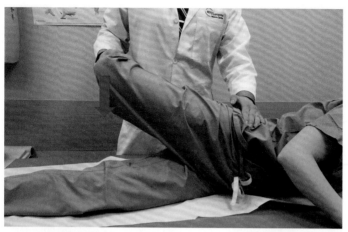

Figure 4-34 Ober's test. Instruct the patient to lie in the lateral decubitus position with the unaffected side against the examination table. Place one hand on the patient's ankle and the other hand over the iliac crest at the lateral hip. Then passively flex the knee to 90 degrees while extending and abducting the hip. Then slowly adduct the hip (Red arrow). Inability to undergo passive hip adduction past the midline may be suggestive of IT band syndrome or an external snapping hip.

Positive Findings: Reproducible pain, locking, or snapping may be suggestive of a posterior labral tear.

The knee and lower leg (Figure 4-35): Begin with the standard inspection. Pay attention to any varus (bowing) or valgus (knock knee) deformity that may be present (Figure 4-36). Continue to inspect for a shiny, hairless, mottled, or discolored appearance of the lower extremity. Evaluate for dilated or varicose veins. Following your assessment, palpate the bony anatomy including the medial and lateral femoral condyles, the patella, the proximal tibial, the tibial tuberosity, and the fibular head. Then, palpate the soft-tissue structures including the quadriceps and patellar tendons, medial and lateral joint lines anteriorly and posteriorly, the MCL and LCL, the IT band (insertion at Gerdy's tubercle), the popliteal fossa (and/or presence of Baker's cyst), and all musculature noting any

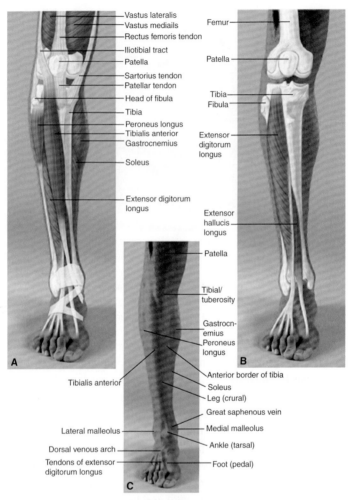

Figure 4-35 **Anatomy of the knee and lower leg**. (From Premkumar K. *The Massage Connection Anatomy and Physiology*. Baltimore, MD: Lippincott Williams & Wilkins; 2004.)

tenderness, crepitus, or edema. Next, assess active and passive ranges of motion (Table 4-15). Next, evaluate muscle strength. Muscles to evaluate:

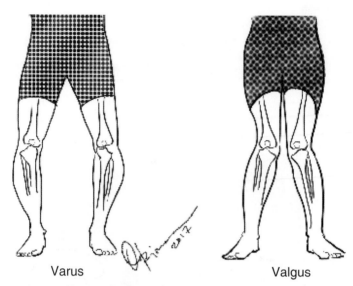

Varus   Valgus

Figure 4-36 Varus and valgus deformities. Varus (bowing) and valgus (knock knee) deformities of the knee.

- Biceps femoris, semitendinosus, semimembranosus, sartorius, gracilis: knee flexion
- Vastus lateralis, intermedius and medialis, rectus femoris: knee extension

Special Tests for the Knee

Evaluation of effusion (Ballottement):

Maneuver: Instruct the patient to slightly flex their knee. With one hand on the suprapatellar pouch, gently push down and toward the patella forcing fluid to accumulate at the central aspect of the joint. Next, gently push down on the patella with your other hand.

Positive Findings: The patella will "bounce" back up or feel as if it is floating once released, which may be suggestive of a sizable effusion.

Evaluation for meniscal injury (Figure 4-37): First, begin by palpating the medial and lateral joint lines with the knee in a slightly

TABLE 4-15	Full Active Range of Motion of the Knee
Motion	**Typical Range (degrees)**
Flexion	130
Extension	0

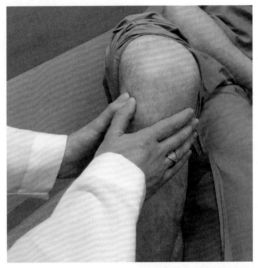

Figure 4-37 Evaluation for meniscal injury. Palpate the medial and lateral joint lines with the knee in a flexed position. Tenderness may be suggestive of underlying meniscal damage.

flexed position. Tenderness may be suggestive of underlying meniscal damage.

McMurray's test: Instruct the patient to lie in a supine position.

Maneuver: To examine the right knee: place your left hand with your index, middle, and ring fingers aligned along the medial joint line. Grasp the right foot with your right hand and fully flex the knee. Extend the knee while externally rotating the tibia and applying a valgus stress.

Positive Findings: Clicking sensation or pain at the knee when the knee is extended may be suggestive of a medial meniscal injury. To assess the lateral meniscus, return the knee to the fully flexed position, extend the knee while internally rotating the tibia and applying a varus stress.

Positive Findings: Clicking sensation or pain at the knee when the knee is extended may be suggestive of a lateral meniscal injury.

Apple Grind Test: Instruct the patient to lie prone.

Maneuver: With one hand, grasp the patient's ankle and with your other hand grasp the midfoot. Flex their knee to 90 degrees. Push down gently while rotating the ankle back and forth.

Positive Findings: Reproducible pain may be suggestive of meniscal pathology.

Evaluation for ligamentous injury: Specific to evaluating for ligamentous injury is learning the mechanism of action that caused the injury (Table 4-16). First, palpate along the ligament for reproducible pain and swelling. The degree of laxity should be noted when examining each ligament (Table 4-17).

Lachman's test—ACL (Figure 4-38): Instruct the patient to completely relax their leg.

Maneuver: Grasp the femur just above the knee with one hand and the tibia with your other. Flex the knee slightly. Pull up sharply on the tibia while stabilizing the femur with your other hand.

Positive Findings: Significant distraction and unrestrained anterior motion of the tibia with a soft end point may be suggestive of ACL pathology (partial or full thickness tear).

Anterior drawer test—ACL (Figure 4-39): Instruct the patient to lie supine with the knee to be *examined* flexed to 90 degrees and their foot flat on the table. Stabilize the foot by gently sitting on it.

Maneuver: With both hands, grasp just distal to the knee, with your fingers around the posterior calf and thumbs meeting along the anterior tibia. Gently pull forward, assessing how much the tibia moves forward relative to the femur.

TABLE 4-16

Ligamentous Injury Mechanisms of Action

Ligament	Most Common Mechanism of Injury	Additional Mechanisms
ACL	Foot planted, extreme rotational force applied	Deceleration impact from a jump, direct force on the lateral knee
PCL	Posterior force on the tibia	Fall on a flexed knee, hyperextension, extreme valgus force
MCL	Direct force on the lateral aspect of the knee while the foot is planted	
LCL	Direct force on the medial aspect of the knee while the foot is planted	

TABLE 4-17

Grading System for Ligament Injuries

Grade	Translation	End Point
1	Fibers stretch, no laxity present	Good
2	Partial tear, mild laxity	Fair
3	Complete tear, significant laxity	Soft

Positive Findings: Unrestrained anterior motion of the tibia and a soft end point may be suggestive of ACL pathology (partial or full thickness tear). Always compare your findings with the contralateral joint if possible.

Pivot shift test (Figure 4-40): Warning: A positive test may illicit significant discomfort for the *patient*. Make them aware before performing. Instruct the patient to lie supine with their knee extended.

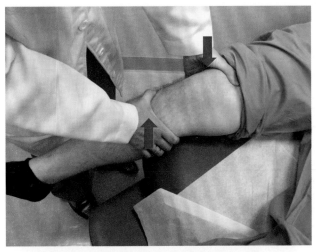

Figure 4-38 Lachman test. After instructing patient to relax their leg, practitioner should slightly flex patient's knee, stabilize their femur with one arm, and pull forward on the tibia with the other arm. Significant anterior tibial motion without hard end point suggestive of ACL pathology. Red arrows demonstrate the vector of force of each hand.

Maneuver: Place your hand under the heel. Internally rotate the foot while placing a valgus directed force at the knee with your other hand. Simultaneously bring the knee from extension to flexion.

Positive Findings: A palpable clunk at 30 degrees of flexion (tibia reducing onto the femur).

Posterior cruciate ligament testing: Instruct the patient to lie supine with the knee to be examined *flexed* to 90 degrees and their foot flat on the table. Stabilize the foot by gently sitting on it.

Maneuver: With both hands, grasp just distal to the knee, with your fingers around the posterior calf and thumbs meeting along the anterior tibia. Gently push backward, assessing how much the tibia moves posteriorly relative to the femur.

Positive Findings: Unrestrained posterior motion of the tibia and a soft end point may be suggestive of PCL pathology

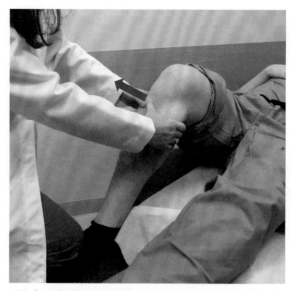

Figure 4-39 **Anterior drawer test.** Instruct patient to lay supine on examination table with knee flexed to 90 degrees and stabilize foot flat on table. Practitioner should wrap their fingers around the posterior calf, just distal to the knee, and gently pull forward while assessing degree of anterior displacement of the tibia. Significant anterior tibial motion without hard end point suggestive of ACL pathology. The red arrow demonstrates the vector of force applied.

(partial or full thickness tear). Always compare your findings with the contralateral joint if possible.

Posterior sag sign (Figure 4-41): Maintaining position similar to that for the anterior/*posterior* drawer tests.

Positive Findings: The tibial tubercle sagging posteriorly relative to the contralateral tibial tuberosity is suggestive of a PCL injury.

Dial test: Instruct the patient to lie prone on the examination table.

Maneuver: Flex the patient's bilateral knees to 30 degrees. Holding the patient's heels or foot, begin externally rotating the leg to maximum ability. Measure the foot–thigh angle bilaterally. Repeat the examination with the knees flexed to 90 degrees.

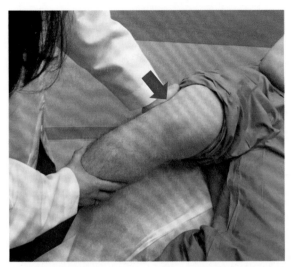

Figure 4-40 **Pivot shift test.** Instruct patient to lay supine on examination table with fully extended, relaxed knee. Practitioner should then hold lower leg in interior rotation while slowly flexing patient's knee and simultaneously providing valgus stress (Red arrow). Palpable "clunk" at 30 to 40 degrees of flexion as tibia reduces onto femur suggestive of ACL pathology and/or other concomitant ligamentous pathology.

Positive Findings: >10 degrees of external rotation in the injured knee compared to the contralateral knee.

MCL testing/Valgus stress (Figure 4-42): Instruct the patient to flex their *knee* to about 30 degrees.

Maneuver: Place one hand along the lateral aspect of the knee and the other hand on the ankle or calf. Push steadily but gently inward on the knee while supplying an opposite force at the calf (valgus stress).

Positive Findings: Joint laxity or complete joint opening is suggestive of MCL partial or complete tears.

Lateral collateral ligament testing: Instruct the patient to flex their knee to about 30 *degrees*.

Maneuver: Place one hand along the medial aspect of the knee and the other hand on the ankle or calf. Push steadily but

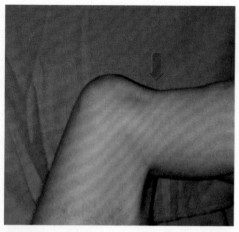

Figure 4-41 Posterior sag sign. Instruct patient to lay supine on examination table with knee flexed. Note posterior sagging of tibial tubercle (Red arrow) which is suggestive of PCL pathology.

gently outward on the knee while supplying an opposite force at the calf.

Positive Findings: Joint laxity or complete joint opening is suggestive of LCL partial or complete tears.

The ankle and foot: Inspect the ankle and foot for deformity (Figure 4-43). Note if the patient has a varus or valgus deformity of the ankle, is flat foot, has a high arch or normal arch (Figure 4-44). If deformity is noted, inspect the patient's shoes for uneven wear. Next, draw attention to the toes. Inspect the nails, skin, and for plantar or dorsal callus. Do they have normal, clawed, hammer, or mallet toes (Figure 4-45)? Inspect plantar surface of the foot for ulcers. This is especially important in diabetics or patients with known peripheral vascular disease.

Next, palpate the bony anatomy: Medial and lateral malleolus, calcaneous, subtler joint, mid foot, forefoot, and toes. Next, palpate soft-tissue structures including: Achilles tendon, the ATFL,

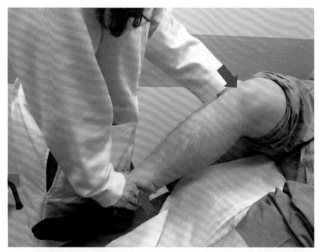

Figure 4-42 MCL test/valgus stress. Instruct the patient to flex their knee to about 30 degrees. Place one hand along the lateral aspect of the knee and the other hand on the ankle or calf. Push steadily but gently inward on the knee while supplying an opposite force at the calf (valgus stress). Joint laxity or complete joint opening is suggestive of MCL partial or complete tears.

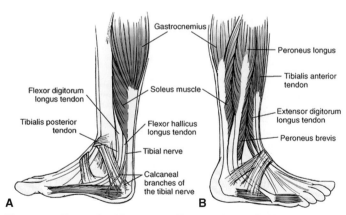

Figure 4-43 Foot and ankle anatomy. (From Hendrickson T. *Massage and Manual Therapy for Orthopedic Conditions.* Philadelphia, PA: Wolters Kluwer; 2009, with permission.)

Normal arch | High arch | Flat arch

Figure 4-44 **Foot arch.** Schematics of normal foot arch, high arch (pes cavus), and flat arch (pes planus).

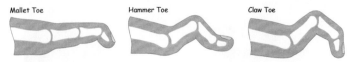

Figure 4-45 **Toe deformities.** Schematics of mallet toe (fixed or flexible deformity at the DIP joint), hammer toe (hyperextension of the MTP, hyperflexion of the PIP), and claw toe (contraction at PIP and DIP joints).

the PTFL, the CFL, and the deltoid ligaments. Next, assess active and passive ranges of motion (Table 4-18). Next, evaluate muscle strength. Muscles to evaluate:

- Gastrocnemius, soleus, tibialis posterior, flexor hallucis longus, flexor digitorum longus: plantar flexion
- Anterior tibialis, extensor hallucis longus, extensor digitorum longus: dorsiflexion
- Anterior and posterior tibialis: inversion
- Peroneus longus and brevis: eversion
- Extensor digitorum longus: MTP extension
- Extensor hallucis longus: great toe extension
- Flexor hallucis longus: great toe flexion, brevis: MTP flexion of great toe
- Flexor digitorum longus: flexion of the four lateral toes
- Flexor digitorum brevis: PIP joint flexion of the four lateral toes

TABLE 4-18 Full Active Range of Motion of the Ankle	
Motion	**Typical Range (degrees)**
Plantar flexion	0–50
Dorsiflexion	0–20
Inversion	0–35
Eversion	0–25

Special Test for the Ankle and Foot

Anterior drawer test: Instruct the patient to sit at the end of the examination table with their *lower* leg hanging off (knee flexed; Figure 4-46).

> **Maneuver:** Stabilize the anterior tibia with one hand. Cupping the heal with your other hand translate the calcaneus forward.
>
> **Positive Findings:** Unrestrained anterior motion of the foot or a clunk at the end point is suggestive of anterior talofibular ligament injury.

Talar tilt test (Figure 4-47): Instruct the patient to sit at the end of the examination table with their lower leg hanging off (knee flexed).

> **Maneuver:** Stabilize the distal leg with one hand. Cupping the heal with your other hand gently invert the foot. Compare with the contralateral ankle.
>
> **Positive Findings:** Excessive ankle inversion or reproducible pain is suggestive of a calcaneofibular ligament injury.
>
> **Maneuver:** Stabilize the distal leg with one hand. Cupping the heal with your other hand gently evert the foot. Compare with the contralateral ankle.
>
> **Positive Findings:** Excessive ankle eversion or reproducible pain is suggestive of a deltoid ligament injury.

Cotton Test:

> **Maneuver:** Stabilize the distal leg with one hand. Place your other hand under the plantar aspect of the foot. Cupping the foot, place your thumb under one malleolus and your

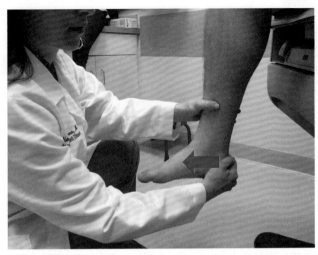

Figure 4-46 Anterior drawer test. Instruct the patient to sit at the end of the examination table with their lower leg hanging off. Stabilize the anterior tibia with one hand. Practitioner should then cup the heel and translate the calcaneus forward (Red arrow). Unrestrained anterior motion of the foot or a clunk at the end point is suggestive of anterior talofibular ligament injury.

middle finger under the other malleolus. Apply a medial, then lateral-directed force on the ankle.

Positive Findings: Excessive translation, soft end point, or reproducible pain may be suggestive of a syndesmotic sprain.

Thompson test (Figure 4-48): Instruct the patient to lie prone on the examination table and flex their knee to 90 degrees.

Maneuver: Squeeze the patient's calf.

Positive Findings: Lack of plantar flexion may be suggestive of Achilles tendon tear.

Sensation Examination

Note if sensation is intact to light touch in the lateral, anterior, and posterior femoral cutaneous, saphenous, peroneal, tibial, and sural nerve distributions (Figure 4-49). Two-point discrimination and monofilament testing should also be performed. If the patient is

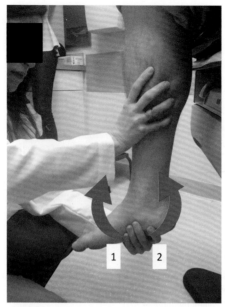

Figure 4-47 **Talar tilt.** Instruct the patient to sit at the end of the examination table with their lower leg hanging off (knee flexed). Stabilize the distal leg with one hand. Cupping the heal with your other hand, gently invert the foot (Red arrow 1). Compare with the contralateral ankle. Excessive ankle inversion or reproducible pain is suggestive of a calcaneofibular ligament injury. Stabilize the distal leg with one hand. Cupping the heal with your other hand gently evert the foot (Red arrow 2). Compare with the contralateral ankle. Excessive ankle eversion or reproducible pain is suggestive of a deltoid ligament injury.

unable to feel the 5.07 monofilament on the sole of their foot, they have lost their protective sense.

Vascular Examination

Be familiar with the lower extremity vasculature (Figure 4-50). First, inspect the extremity: Does it appear pink, perfused and feel warm? Or is it cool to the touch, dusky and with pallor? Has a portion of the limb become necrotic? Assess areas of pressure: the lateral aspect of the foot, head of the first metatarsal, the heal, medial and lateral

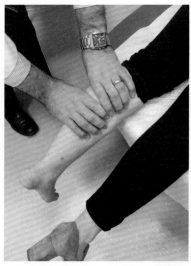

Figure 4-48 **Thompson's test.** Instruct patient to lay prone on examination table. Practitioner should then squeeze calf muscle. Lack of plantar flexion suggestive of Achilles tendon tear.

malleoli, bony prominences of the toes. Assess for femoral, popliteal, posterior tibial, and dorsalis pedis pulses and grade accordingly. If unable to palpate pulses, use a Doppler ultrasonic probe for pulse detection. Also, comment on capillary refill.

IV. IMAGING AND DIAGNOSTIC TESTING

Plain Radiographic Imaging

An accurate diagnosis that may be identified by X-ray is best achieved when two quality orthogonal views are obtained. Most commonly these views are anteroposterior and lateral views. These images must be appropriately penetrated, without overlying or obstructing objects in view, and centered on the joint or bone of interest. Some injuries may require further evaluation with additional views such as an oblique view or a view specific to identifying or ruling out the suspected injury. *Important*: all diaphyseal fractures require

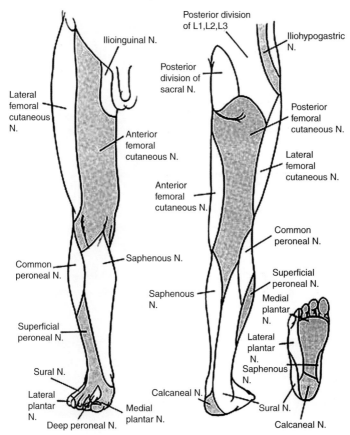

Figure 4-49 Cutaneous innervation of lower extremity. (From Brown DL, Borschel GH, Levi B. *Michigan Manual of Plastic Surgery*. Philadelphia, PA: Wolters Kluwer; 2014, with permission.)

orthogonal X-rays of the joints above and below the injury to assess for additional fractures or joint dislocations.

Computerized Tomography

Other injuries require more advanced imaging for an evaluation or diagnosis. Specifically, complex fractures, suspected tumors,

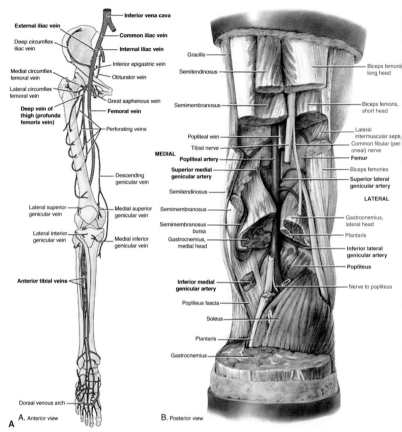

Figure 4-50 **Lower extremity vasculature.** (From Rubin P, Hansen JT. *TNM Staging Atlas with Oncoanatomy.* Philadelphia, PA: Wolters Kluwer; 2012, with permission.)

spinal injuries, and pelvic injuries may necessitate a CT scan with or without 3D reconstruction. This imaging modality produced a more detailed 2D image that is sensitive for subtle and nondisplaced fractures and aids in the assessment of fracture healing, articular surface distortion, and the diagnosis of fracture nonunions. Often, CT imaging is utilized in operative planning for articular fractures. 3D reconstructive images, which further define the characteristics of an injury, can be generated without additional radiation exposure (Figure 4-51).

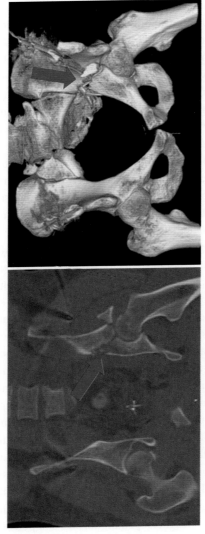

Figure 4-51 2D CT scan with 3D reconstruction. 2D CT scan on left demonstrating left-sided acetabular fracture with 3D reconstruction on right. Red arrow identifies the fracture line.

Magnetic Resonance Imaging

MRI is often indicated to evaluate soft-tissue structures such as ligaments, tendons, cartilage, and muscles for acute traumatic injuries or structural abnormalities. It is considered the gold standard for diagnosing meniscal and ligamentous injuries of the knee as well as rotator cuff and labral tears in the shoulder. MRI may also be utilized to evaluate other conditions such as osteonecrosis, tumors, spinal disc herniation or degeneration, inflammatory disease, or congenital abnormalities. MRI is more sensitive in detecting microfractures, stress fractures, and bone contusions or those not evident on X-ray examination.

Important: all patients must be screened for implanted devices and external metal objects. Fracture hardware and joint implants are not a contraindication to MRI because the metals used in these materials are not magnetic. Exercise caution in evaluating patients for pacemakers, heart valve replacements, cochlear implants, implanted pumps (insulin), surgical clips (aneurysm), retained GSW, or wire mesh. For patients for whom you are evaluating an area close to implanted orthopaedic hardware, make note to the radiologist to implement the metal artifact reduction sequences when performing their examination. This protocol will help reduce metal artifact and improve the quality of the images obtained.

Also, some patients may express concerns regarding claustrophobia and the ability to complete an MRI examination. A prescription for a one-time dose of an anxiolytic may be indicated in this situation. For example, Alprazolam 5 mg tablet. Sig: 1 tab po, 30 minutes prior to examination. Additionally, confirm that your patient is capable of lying flat and still for up to an hour.

Regarding all imaging, it is important that you do not base treatment recommendations solely off of the radiologists' reading without personally viewing and interpreting the images. Remember, that the radiologist is another provider on the patient's health care team and your colleague. If you are unsure of a personal finding or their interpretation of the imaging, speak to the radiologist directly for clarification.

When ordering CT or MRI, an IV contrast would enhance your examination; first check the patient's GFR to confirm if it is >30 mL/min/1.73 m². If the patient's GFR is <30 mL/min/1.73 m², it is advised to avoid administering contrast because of the risk of contrast-induced nephropathy. If the examination necessitates IV contrast, follow these guidelines to reduce the risk of CIN:

- Increasing the amount of time between contrast-enhanced examinations.
- Decreasing the total volume of contrast administered.
- Initiate periprocedural volume expansion therapy—IV hydration with an isotonic fluid (Lactated Ringer's or 0.9% NS) at 100 mL/hour, for 6 to 12 hours prior to contrast administration and for 4 to 12 hours after completion of the examination.
- Avoid all other nephrotoxins.
- Administer Mucomyst (*N*-acetylcysteine) po, 600 mg bid on the day before and the day of the contrast imaging study.

Ultrasound

Ultrasound (US) imaging is a safe and noninvasive imaging technique that provides real-time data and high-resolution images (Chapter 1, Figure 1-9). It is often utilized to evaluate soft-tissue pathology including masses, fluid collections, tendon injuries/rupture, tenosynovitis, ligamentous injuries, congenital hip disorders in children, and carpal tunnel syndrome. US can identify the presence of calcifications as well as foreign bodies. Additionally, US imaging aids in therapeutic interventions by improving the accuracy of joint or cyst aspiration/injection procedures. US imaging also allows for dynamic assessments, which may be helpful in determining joint and tendon movements as well as stability. Because US imaging is noninvasive, does not emit ionizing radiation, is without contraindications similar to MRI, and is cost-effective, it is an excellent imaging modality that may be indicated for repeat imaging.

Dual-Energy X-ray Absorptiometry

DEXA scanning is an imaging modality that utilizes a small dose of ionizing radiation to evaluate bone loss. It is the gold standard for diagnosing osteoporosis and evaluating a patient's risk for future fragility fractures. DEXA scans are indicated as a screening tool for women ≥65 and men ≥70 years of age. In the orthopaedic patient, someone who has experienced 2+ fragility fractures prior to the above-mentioned ages warrant a DEXA scan. Other risk factors for osteoporosis include premature menopause (<45 years), women discontinuing estrogen supplements, a history of eating disorder, patients who received steroid treatment for >3 months in 1 year's time, patients who are on long-term warfarin, heparin, aromatase inhibitors, chemotherapy, phenytoin, or phenobarbital.

Electromyography

Electromyography (EMG) studies are indicated for the evaluation of conditions affecting lower motor neurons. There are two types of EMG studies: intramuscular EMG (more specific assessment) and surface EMG. EMG studies evaluate the presence, size, and shape of an action potential generating a waveform, which is then translated into information regarding the capability of a muscle to respond to nervous stimulation. The electrical activity is mapped by an oscilloscope to reveal an innervated muscle without deficit, a partially denervated muscle, a completely denervated muscle, nerve regeneration, a partial or complete nerve lesion, or myotonia. Advise your patient that for an intramuscular EMG to be performed, needle electrodes are inserted into the muscle, which may cause discomfort similar to receiving an injection.

Nerve conduction studies may be utilized to determine the motor conduction velocity. Normal motor velocities in the upper extremities are >45 m/s and in the lower extremities >40 m/s. Velocities are affected by temperature, that is, vascularity, and the location of the nerve segment being evaluated (distal vs. proximal). Normal sensory nerve conduction velocities in the upper extremity are >35 m/s (in the wrist to elbow segment). Sensory studies are strongly positive when there is an absent response.

These examinations are often utilized in patients with post-traumatic, postsurgical, or primary motor or sensory deficits. Ordering an EMG nerve conduction study at the patient's initial appointment will document their presenting deficit, which can later be compared to follow-up examinations to assess for regenerative nerve activity.

New patients that are indicated for surgery may require laboratory evaluation and further diagnostic workup for medical clearance. Some of this will be completed by the preadmission testing team; however, you may order some tests to expedite the process (Table 4-19). Additionally, for patients that may experience high-volume blood loss, a type and screen and/or cross should also be ordered. If you plan to screen for any further vitamin deficiencies or conditions, provide your patient with these orders as well, so all laboratory studies can be completed in one setting.

V. PLAN OF CARE

If you have collected all the necessary data to evaluate your patient's injury or condition, educate your patient on all treatment options available with supportive data regarding expected outcomes for each option. Have a detailed discussion regarding risks, benefits, and alternatives to each of the options. In a collaborative effort with your patient and supervising physician, taking current health status, previous level of function and independence, and future goals into account, determine which treatment recommendation will give your patient the best possible outcome. During this discussion, empower the patient with shared decision-making to ensure that they are comfortable with their plan of care. If further testing or consultation is required prior to making final recommendations, explain to the patient why this additional information is valuable and how it may impact the recommendations made. You can then outline the necessary next steps for gathering this information. Refer to Chapters

TABLE
4-19

Preoperative Diagnosis–Based Investigations Before Elective Surgery[6]

CBC	Serum Creatinine and Electrolytes	Blood Glucose	ECG	Chest X-rays	Coagulation Studies
Major surgery	Kidney disease	Diabetes or family history of diabetes	Cardiac disease	Chronic lung disease	Liver disease
Neonates	Hypertension	Obesity	Hypertension	Active/previous smoker	Renal dysfunctions
Males >70 Females >45	Diabetes	Stroke	Diabetes	Radiation therapy	Family history of a bleeding disorder
Chronic renal, liver, or lung disease	Poor nutritional states	Poor nutritional states	Poor nutritional states	Aortic aneurysm	On anticoagulant medication
Anemia	Stroke	Steroid use	Stroke	Cardiomegaly	
Malignancy	Medications: Digoxin, diuretics, steroids, chemotherapy	Cushing's or Addison's disease	Medications: Digoxin, diuretics, steroids, chemotherapy		
Poor nutritional states					
Vascular aneurysms					

6 and 7 for further information regarding operative and nonoperative management, goals of treatment, and outcome expectations.

Timeline

Present a generalized timeline for further evaluation, treatment, and recovery. This will help prepare your patient for the upcoming days, weeks, or months of treatment and set expectations for recovery. Things to consider:

Advanced Imaging

Is further imagining necessary? If so, is prior authorization required? Prior authorization can take anywhere from 1 hour to 1+ weeks to obtain. Several insurance carriers may require additional clinical information despite receiving official history and physical examination notes from support staff. It is not uncommon for an initial request to be denied, then requiring a peer-to-peer discussion with a physician reviewer from the insurance company. Formal letters explaining need for advanced imaging may also be required for further review. Make your patient aware that often prior authorization can be obtained within 1 to 2 days, but may take up to a week.

Once authorization is received, the examination may be schedule by the patient directly or by support staff. Be familiar with the average wait times for several facilities in your area. Many urban hospital systems may be able to accommodate same-day scheduling, whereas more rural locations may not have availability for over a week for routine imaging.

Once imaging is completed, the official radiology report is often received or available within 24 hours. If imaging is performed at an outside facility where you do not have privileges to access results, inform your patient it is necessary that they request a CD or file with imaging to view. They may also request for the images to be electronically transmitted or mailed directly to your practice. It may take up to a week to obtain actual images. Remind your patient that until you directly view the study, a final recommendation regarding treatment cannot be made.

Lab Work

Again, length of wait for an appointment or results depends on facility. If the blood draw is completed at a lab within your institution, results are often accessible within several hours depending on the test ordered. If the blood draw is completed at an unaffiliated outpatient lab, results are typically received between 1 and 7 days. Establish an office policy for informing patients of their results.

Recommendation

If your office is equipped with an electronic medical record system with a patient portal for access, encourage your patients to enroll. This will grant the patient real-time access to their results, and allow direct communication between the patient and provider via the portal regarding any concerns. If this application is not available, it is recommended that you inform the patient that you will initiate communication once the office has received their results. The policy aids to eliminate multiple incoming phone calls to support staff questioning if the results have been received.

Consultation

In the event that you feel your patient would benefit from another physician or specialist consult, inform your patient of the rationale supporting the need for this consult and provide them with the name and contact information of the specialist. To help expedite this process, your office support staff can aid in setting up their initial appointment or providing a referral if required. If for some reason, this health care provider is not in network with your patients' insurance plan, provide at minimum two other recommendations. Following your patients' appointment, it may take 1 to 2 days to receive communication from the health care professional regarding their recommendations. Discuss this time frame with your patient and remind them that you are working in conjunction with the consultant to provide the best possible health care.

At the end of *every* patient encounter, ask, "Do you have any further questions or concerns that I can address today?" This reassures the patient that you are committed to their care and will take the time necessary to clarify any confusion. As you walk the patient out, directly communicate to support staff the plan of care for the patient. Below are some topics to highlight:

- Timeline for their follow-up appointment and which health care provider they should be scheduled with (PA or surgeon).
- Medication prescriptions—if prior authorization is necessary or if medications were E-scribed.
- Therapy prescriptions and recommendation for therapy facilities.
- Laboratory prescriptions and recommendation for lab sites.
- Orthopaedic device prescriptions and if prior authorization is necessary.
- Advanced imaging prescriptions—assistance with scheduling the examination and prior authorization if necessary.
- Physician referral paperwork and face sheet with contact information. If a very timely appointment is required, request your staff reaches out to their office on the patient's behalf.
- PAT and surgical scheduling information.

REFERENCES

1. 2013 Statistical Profile of Certified PAs. NCCPA. https://www.nccpa .net/Upload/PDFs/2013StatisticalProfileofCertifiedPhysicianAssis-tants-AnAnnualReportoftheNCCPA.pdf. Accessed January 10, 2016.
2. Final Update Summary: Alcohol Misuse: Screening and Behavioral Counseling Interventions in Primary Care. U.S. Preventive Services Task Force. http://www.uspreventiveservicestaskforce.org/Page/ Document/UpdateSummaryFinal/alcohol-misuse-screening-and-behavioral-counseling-interventions-in-primary-care?ds=1&s=alcohol. Accessed January 20, 2016.
3. Examination of the hand and wrist. iKnowledge. http://clinicalgate .com/1-examination-of-the-hand-and-wrist/. Accessed September 4, 2016.

4. Moore D. Neck & upper extremity spine exam—spine. *Orthobullets.* http://www.orthobullets.com/spine/2001/neck-and-upper-extremity-spine-exam. Accessed September 6, 2016.

5. Moore D. Lower extremity spine & Neuro exam—spine. *Orthobullets.* http://www.orthobullets.com/spine/2002/lower-extremity-spine-and-neuro-exam. Accessed September 6, 2016.

6. Kumar A, Srivastava U. Role of routine laboratory investigations in preoperative evaluation. *J Anesthesiol Clin Pharmacol.* 2011;27(2):174-179.

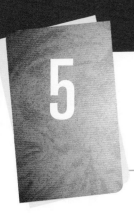

ORTHOPAEDIC SURGICAL PATIENTS: AN OVERVIEW

Ariana Lott and Kenneth A. Egol

I. HIP AND KNEE OSTEOARTHRITIS

Arthritis, the inflammation of one or more joints, can occur secondary to the result of trauma, infection, or age-related degeneration. Arthritis is the single most common cause of disability among older adults, with 40% of those over the age of 65 having symptomatic hip or knee arthritis.[1] No matter the cause, pain secondary to arthritis is usually progressive and can lead to a significant decrease in one's ability to engage in daily activities and therefore in one's overall quality of life. Although less common in patients under the age of 45, the incidence of osteoarthritis increases with each decade of life as shown in the incidence rates of hip and knee arthritis (Table 5-1). Treatments aim to reduce pain, improve quality of life, and prevent further joint damage. First-line treatments for patients with arthritis include nonsteroidal anti-inflammatory drugs (NSAIDs; Table 5-2), physical therapy, and weight loss for patients with BMI ≥ 25.[2,3] Although the evidence on bracing for patients with knee arthritis is inconclusive, some patients may benefit from a valgus bracing for isolated medial compartment osteoarthritis to reduce pressure on the medial compartment of the knee.[4] In patients that have continued pain despite these treatments, intra-articular glucocorticoid and/or hyaluronic acid injections are recommended. These injections reach their maximum effect at 2 weeks and can relieve pain for up to 6 months.[5] Injections can be repeated every 3 months; however, even with continued administration, benefits may plateau after 2 years of therapy.

| TABLE 5-1 | Annual Incidence Rates (Per 1,000 Person-Years) of Symptomatic Hip and Knee Arthritis by Age[17,18] |

Age (years)	Symptomatic Hip OA	Symptomatic Knee OA
45-54	8	18
55-64	16	24
65-74	28	26
≥75	28	34

| TABLE 5-2 | List of Nonsteroidal Anti-Inflammatory Drugs Listed Alphabetically |

Nonsteroidal Anti-Inflammatory Drug	Mechanism of Action
1. Aspirin	Irreversible COX-1 and COX-2 inhibitor
2. Celecoxib (Celebrex)	Selective COX-2 inhibitor
3. Ibuprofen (Motrin, Advil)	Reversible COX-1 and COX-2 inhibitor
4. Indomethacin (Indocin)	Reversible COX-1 and COX-2 inhibitor
5. Ketorolac (Toradol)	Reversible COX-1 and COX-2 inhibitor
6. Naproxen (Aleve, Naprosyn)	Reversible COX-1 and COX-2 inhibitor
7. Oxaprozin (Daypro)	Reversible COX-1 and COX-2 inhibitor

If these nonoperative treatments fail to control the pain and disability of arthritis, arthroplasty, surgical replacement of the articular surface of a joint with an artificial prosthesis, is indicated. Particularly due to people living active lives for longer periods of time, such joint replacements have become the most common orthopaedic procedures performed in the United States.[6] However,

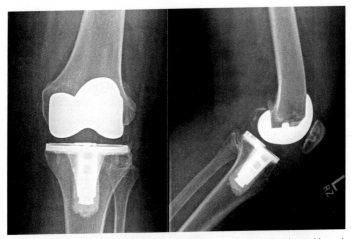

Figure 5-1 Radiograph of a total knee arthroplasty. Anteroposterior and lateral radiographs of the left knee demonstrating cemented total knee replacement.

arthroplasty procedures should only be performed when the patient and physician feel that the pain in the affected joint is debilitating and that no other treatment will provide satisfactory relief.

The most common arthroplasty procedure is the total knee replacement (Figure 5-1), with over 700,000 operations performed yearly in the United States making it the third most performed operation.[6] The knee joint comprises three compartments—lateral, medial, and patellofemoral. Damage to the cartilage lining in any of these compartments can cause severe pain with weight bearing that is often aggravated by climbing stairs or simply going from sitting to standing. As the damage continues, patients may develop bowing deformities or complain of instability. The cause of this damage to the cartilage lining is usually secondary to changes associated with osteoarthritis, but may also be seen in rheumatoid arthritis, avascular necrosis, or at the end stage of some congenital deformities. The majority of knee replacements performed are total knee replacements in that they involve resurfacing all three compartments of the joint: the lateral, medial, and patellofemoral compartments. However, in the case of isolated lateral or medial compartment disease, a unicompartmental arthroplasty may be performed. Possible complications with total knee replacements include patellofemoral maltracking, component loosening, and infection.

Another common arthroplasty procedure is the hip replacement (Figure 5-2A and B), with over 450,000 hip replacements performed yearly in the United States making it the fourth most performed operation.[6] The hip joint is composed of the articulation between the acetabulum of the pelvis and the femoral head. It is when the cartilage lining this articular surface is disrupted that patients

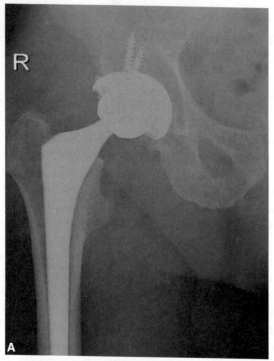

Figure 5-2 A: Radiograph of total hip arthroplasty. Anteroposterior (AP) radiograph of the right hip demonstrating noncemented total hip arthroplasty. **B: Radiograph of hemiarthroplasty.** AP radiograph of the pelvis demonstrating cemented unipolar hemiarthroplasty.

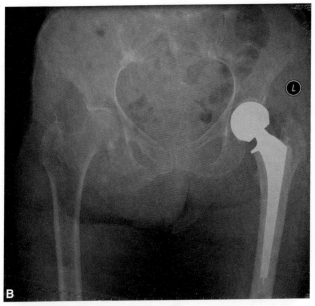

Figure 5-2 (*continued*)

complain of discomfort. Patients with arthritis of the hip may complain of pain in the groin, outer thigh, knee, and/or buttock. They often complain of pain with walking distances and may even have a limp. Although osteoarthritis is the most common cause for hip arthroplasty, other causes include rheumatoid arthritis, avascular necrosis, developmental dysplasia of the hip (DDH), post-traumatic arthritis, and fracture. There are two types of hip arthroplasty: in total hip arthroplasty, both the femoral head and acetabular lining are replaced (Figure 5-2A); in hemiarthroplasty, only the femoral head is replaced keeping the native acetabulum (Figure 5-2B). Although hip replacements are very well-tolerated procedures, possible complications include hip dislocation, periprosthetic joint infection, thromboembolic disease, and periprosthetic fracture (Figure 5-3). Although newer surgical approaches may decrease the number of patients sustaining hip dislocation, the incidence of such

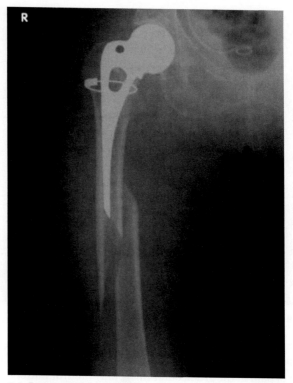

Figure 5-3 **Periprosthetic hip fracture.** Anteroposterior radiograph of the right hip demonstrating periprosthetic fracture below a noncemented hemiarthroplasty.

complications is cited at 1% to 3%, with 70% of those dislocations occurring within the first month.[7] Two of the more significant causes of dislocation are hardware loosening and infection.

II. HAND AND WRIST INJURIES

Orthopaedic surgeons as well as hand specialists see patients with conditions and trauma related to the fingers, hand, and wrist. The anatomy of this area of the human body is complex, with 27 bones in the hand and 8 carpal bones in the wrist plus connective tendons and supportive nerves, all of which allow people to normally engage in a wide range of precise motion. It also creates the opportunity for many different injuries.

The most common fractures in the hand and wrist are distal radius fractures (Figure 5-4). Such fractures can result from high-energy injuries in the young or lower-energy injuries (such as falls) in the elderly. These fractures are often associated with distal ulna or radioulnar joint injuries. Half of these fractures are intra-articular and may require surgical fixation. Although fractures of the distal radius are the most common, there is a substantial incidence of fractures of other parts of the hand and wrist (as shown in Table 5-3). For patients over the age of 65, carpal bones are other common types of hand/wrist fractures. The most common carpal bone injuries are scaphoid fractures, typically caused by a patient catching

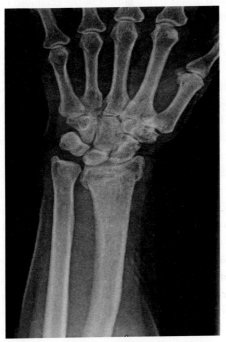

Figure 5-4 Radiograph of a distal radius fracture. Anteroposterior radiograph of the right wrist demonstrating displaced intra-articular distal radius fracture.

TABLE 5-3	Distribution of Hand and Wrist Fractures by Anatomic Site[19]

Anatomic Site	Percentage of Fractures (%)
Radius and/or ulna	44
Phalanx/phalanges	23
Metacarpal(s)	18
Carpal	14
Multiple hand bones	1

his/her fall with an outstretched hand. Although most of these fractures can be treated nonoperatively, some do require surgery because the tenuous blood supply of the scaphoid bone creates an increased risk of nonunion and avascular necrosis, potentially leading to later arthritis (Figure 5-5).

Nerve injuries of the hand and wrist are also common with compressive neuropathies responsible for most of these injuries. In these conditions, direct mechanical pressure on the nerve results in such symptoms as pain, numbness, and sometimes muscle weakness. These compressive neuropathies can occur in the three major nerves of the upper extremity: median nerve, ulnar nerve, and radial nerve (Figure 5-6). The resulting symptoms depend on the damaged nerve and the location of this injury. Median nerve compression is the most common compressive neuropathy seen in the hand and wrist. Median nerve compression can result in carpal tunnel syndrome (CTS), anterior interosseous syndrome, and pronator syndrome. CTS is the most common of these, with an incidence of approximately 375 per 100,000 person-years.[8] This is caused by compression of the median nerve, most often as the nerve travels under the transverse carpal ligament in the carpal tunnel of the wrist. These patients will particularly complain of neuropathic symptoms on the palmar side of the three most radial fingers and the radial side of the fourth digit, with symptoms worse at night. Although risk factors for CTS include obesity,

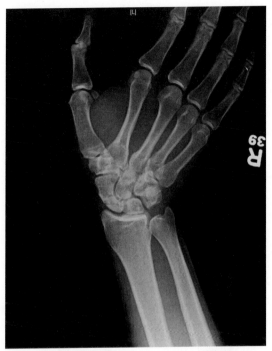

Figure 5-5 **Radiograph of nonunion of scaphoid.** Anteroposterior radiograph of right wrist in ulnar deviation demonstrating nonunion of a scaphoid fracture.

pregnancy, and diabetes, the most common form of CTS in adults is idiopathic. Anterior interosseous syndrome presents as grip and pinch weakness, with patients classically unable to make an "OK" sign due to an inability to flex their thumb and index finger. This results from compression of the anterior interosseous nerve (AIN), the last motor branch of the median nerve, most often under the deep head of the pronator teres. Unlike the other common median nerve neuropathies, patients with this syndrome have no sensory deficits because the AIN has no cutaneous sensory branches. The third median nerve syndrome is pronator syndrome, resulting from compression of the median nerve at the elbow. This results in pain over the volar forearm and neuropathic symptoms on the palmar

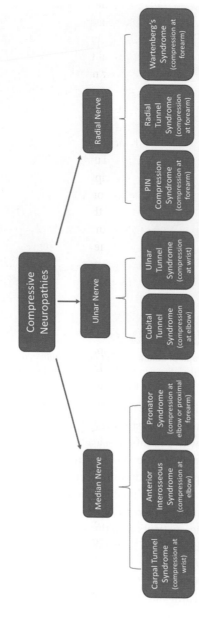

Figure 5-6 Compressive neuropathies. Schematic of hand/wrist compressive neuropathies.

side of the three radial fingers and the radial side of the fourth digit. Unlike CTS, these neuropathic sensory changes extend into the palm. Ulnar nerve neuropathies include cubital tunnel syndrome and ulnar tunnel syndrome. Cubital tunnel syndrome is typically caused by compression of the ulnar nerve between the two heads of the flexor carpi ulnaris muscle. Symptoms include paresthesias of the fifth finger, ulnar side of the fourth finger, and ulnar side of the dorsum of the hand exacerbated with elbow flexion in addition to weakness of the intrinsic hand muscles resulting in decreased grip and pinch strength. The second ulnar nerve neuropathy, ulnar tunnel syndrome, results from compression of the ulnar nerve in Guyon's canal located at the base of the ulnar side of the palm. Symptoms include paresthesias of the palmar aspect of the fifth finger and the ulnar side of the fourth finger; however, patients should not have any symptoms in the dorsum of the hand. Similar to cubital tunnel syndrome, patients may also experience weakness of the intrinsic hand muscles resulting in decreased grip and pinch strength. Radial nerve neuropathies include posterior interosseous nerve (PIN) compression syndrome, radial tunnel syndrome, and Wartenberg's syndrome. These are much rarer than median nerve and ulnar nerve compressive neuropathies. PIN compression syndrome is due to compression of the PIN that innervates the extensor muscles. Compression most commonly occurs at the proximal edge of the supinator, also known as the Arcade of Frohse. Patients complain of pain in the forearm and wrist and weakness with wrist extension. Radial tunnel syndrome also results from compression of the posterior interosseous nerve; however, patients only complain of aching pain in the dorsoradial forearm. There will be no sensory or motor deficits. Wartenberg's syndrome results from compression of the superficial sensory radial nerve between the brachioradialis and extensor carpi radialis longus tendons. Patients complain of paresthesias and pain over the dorsoradial hand. Physical examination of these patients will reveal no motor weakness.

The nerves of the hand, including the digital nerves of each finger can also be injured by laceration. These nerves are purely sensory nerves and provide protective sensation. Injury to these digital nerves results in finger numbness. If a digital nerve is injured proximal to the crease created when the distal interphalangeal (DIP) is flexed, it should be surgically repaired. However, when the injury occurs distal to this crease, the nerve branches are too small to repair. With these injuries, sensation typically returns with time.

The most common tendon injuries in the hand are tendinopathies in which the tendons become compressed and inflamed because of the thickening of tendon sheaths. Trigger finger is one of the most prevalent types of tendinopathy, with the classic patient being a woman over the age of 50. Patients with trigger finger (also known as stenosing tenosynovitis) present with the inability to flex or extend one or more of their fingers (most often their ring finger). Other common forms of tendinopathy include De Quervain's tenosynovitis which occurs when the tendons at the base of the thumb become swollen and inflamed. These patients have pain when making a fist, gripping an object, and/or turning the wrist.

The tendons of the hand can also be injured as a result of trauma. There are two groups of tendons in the hand, flexor tendons and extensor tendons. Flexor tendons assist in flexing or bending the fingers, whereas extensor tendons assist in straightening the fingers. Flexor tendon injuries often occur as a result of palm lacerations. Patients will present with the inability to flex one or more digits and, with these injuries, it is important to test both DIP and proximal interphalangeal flexion. If these injuries involve less than 60% of the tendon, wound care and nonoperative treatment may be elected; however, if the injury involves a greater proportion of the tendon, surgery is required to regain normal function. One example of a flexor tendon injury is "Jersey Finger," which refers to an avulsion injury of the flexor digitorum profundus from its insertion at the base of the distal phalanx. This usually occurs at the ring finger. Extensor tendon injuries result from lacerations to the dorsum of the hand or trauma such as finger jamming. Most of these injuries can be treated with splinting; however, if greater than 50% of the tendon has been torn, tendon repair is necessary. One example of an extensor tendon injury is "Mallet Finger," which refers to an injury of the extensor digitorum tendon distal to the DIP joint. Patients will present with the injured fingertip rested at 45 degrees of flexion and will be unable to actively extend the DIP joint. Most of these injuries can be treated nonoperatively using extension splinting of the DIP joint for 6 to 8 weeks.

Lastly, tendon injuries can result from infection. Infections of the surrounding tendon synovial sheath can be due to direct penetrating trauma or due to spread from felon (infected fingertip) or surrounding septic joints. *Staphylococcus aureus* is the most common organism responsible for these infections. Patients will complain of pain and swelling typically localized to the palmar aspect of one digit. The physical examination of these patients will be notable for erythema and the four Kanavel signs in the affected finger: (1) flexed posture, (2) tenderness to palpation, (3) pain with passive extension, and (4) swelling.

III. ATHLETIC INJURIES

Sports medicine orthopaedics involves the treatment of injuries sustained by people engaged in physical activity, whether as novices (including the so-called weekend-warriors) or as professional athletes. Many of these injuries are acute and involve the knee such as anterior cruciate ligament (ACL) and meniscal tears (Figure 5-7), whereas others are overuse injuries such as stress fractures. The most common injuries requiring an orthopaedic sports specialist are shoulder and knee injuries.

Common shoulder injuries include rotator cuff pathology, shoulder impingement syndrome, and shoulder instability. The rotator cuff is a group of four tendons that are important for both stability and movement of the shoulder. Rotator cuff disease can be the result of either chronic degenerative tears from performing repetitive overhead activities such as throwing or acute tears from a fall causing a shoulder dislocation. The most commonly injured

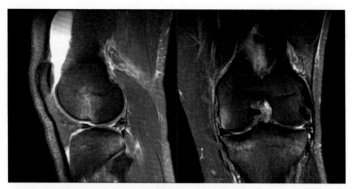

Figure 5-7 **MRI of anterior cruciate ligament (ACL) tear with "kissing contusions."** Sagittal and coronal T2-weighted images demonstrating complete ACL tear with bony contusion of medial femoral condyles and medial tibial plateau (as demonstrated with red arrows).

tendon is the supraspinatus tendon causing patients to have difficulty with abduction of their arm (Figure 5-8). Shoulder impingement syndrome is due to the narrowing of the space between the acromion and the rotator cuff muscles, resulting in pain when one raises his/her arm to shoulder height. It is also a risk factor for the development of rotator cuff tendinopathy because the impingement causes inflammation of the tendons leading to tears.

Shoulder instability is another common shoulder injury. The mechanism for an anterior dislocation is an anterior force with the arm in abduction and external rotation (Figure 5-9). Recurrent shoulder instability due to excessive translation of the humeral head over the glenoid rim results in continued pain due to translation of the humeral head on the glenoid. These dislocations are associated with labrum injuries as well as bone defects. Labrum and cartilage injuries include Bankart lesions, which involve avulsion injuries of the anterior labrum from the anterior glenoid (Figure 5-10). Common bone defects include a Hill–Sachs deficit and a bony Bankart lesion. Hill–Sachs deficits refer to posterolateral humeral head compression fractures, and bony Bankart lesions refer to fractures of the inferior anterior glenoid.

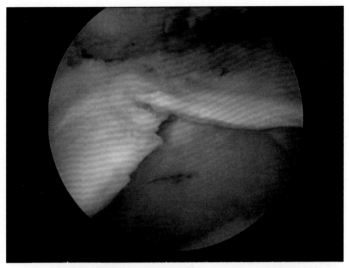

Figure 5-8. Rotator cuff tear. Arthroscopic image demonstrating rotator cuff tear.

Knee injuries can be separated into ligamentous injuries, meniscal injuries, cartilage injuries, and extensor mechanism injuries. Ligamentous injuries include tears of the ACL and the posterior cruciate ligament (PCL), as well as tears of the medial collateral ligament and the lateral collateral ligament. ACL injuries commonly result from noncontact pivoting injuries; they are far more common in women than in men (with a ratio of 2:1). Athletes suffering an ACL injury will often hear a "pop" noise and complain of immediate swelling due to hemarthrosis. Examination of these patients is notable for increased anterior translation of the tibia on the femur. ACL reconstruction is indicated in patients who would like to return to high-demand sports. Surgical intervention is also recommended for patients with multiple ligamentous injuries and continued knee instability. PCL injuries, although less common than ACL injuries, are often undiagnosed in acute knee injuries. They most commonly result from direct blows to the proximal tibia with the knee flexed and from hyperextension. Patients sustaining PCL tears complain of posterior

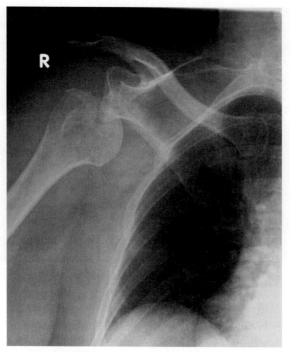

Figure 5-9 Radiograph of anterior shoulder dislocation. Anteroposterior radiograph of right shoulder demonstrating anterior inferior shoulder dislocation.

knee pain and instability with posterior translation of the tibia on the femur. Reconstruction is indicated in combined ligamentous injuries and some isolated PCL injuries with an associated avulsion fracture. Many isolated PCL injuries can be managed nonoperatively.

Most sports-related knee surgeries are performed for medial and/or lateral meniscal tears. Because the medial meniscus is less mobile than the lateral meniscus, medial meniscal injuries are generally more common than lateral meniscal injuries (Figure 5-11). However, in acute ACL injuries, lateral meniscal tears are more common. Meniscal injuries can be acute and secondary to traumatic twisting injuries or chronic as in the case of degenerative

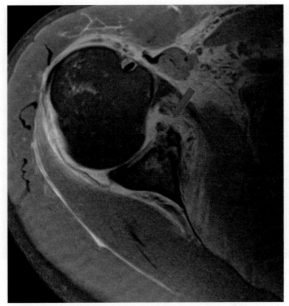

Figure 5-10 MRI of Bankart lesion. T2-weighted image with red arrow pointing to disruption in anterior capsuloligamentous complex.

meniscal tears more commonly seen in older patients. Patients with ACL-deficient knees are at a higher risk for meniscal injuries and long-term osteoarthritis. These patients present with joint line tenderness, difficulty squatting, and knee locking and clicking symptoms.[9] Surgery is indicated in patients who have continued symptoms and swelling and who have large complex tears, especially those that interact with the articular cartilage.

Articular cartilage injuries of the knee range from single lesions to diffuse cartilage damage resulting from acute trauma or chronic large impact forces to the knee. Partial-thickness lesions that do not reach subchondral bone have no ability to heal as they are avascular. In contrast, full-thickness lesions can fill in with a fibro-cartilagenous scar.[9(pp1134-1148)] These lesions tend to occur on the femoral condyle and the patella. Lesions on the femoral condyle are

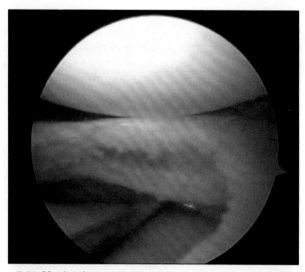

Figure 5-11 **Meniscal tear.** Arthroscopic image demonstrating radial tear of medial meniscus.

typically due to chronic ACL tears and osteochondritis dissecans lesions, whereas patellar lesions are often seen following patella dislocations. For patients with mild symptoms, anti-inflammatories, physical therapy, and weight loss can help reduce pain. However, as cartilage injuries have limited healing capacity, surgery is often required for more severe lesions. For patients with femoral lesions, microfracture, osteochondral autograft/allograft transfer, or autologous chondrocyte implantation can be performed in combination with addressing malalignment, ligament instability, and meniscal injuries. For patients with patellofemoral lesions, microfracture or osteochondral autograft transfer or autologous chondrocyte implantation can be performed supplemented with addressing patellofemoral maltracking and malalignment.[9(pp1134-1148)]

Lastly, extensor mechanism injuries result from quadriceps tendon ruptures and patella tendon ruptures. Quadriceps tendon ruptures are more common than patella tendon ruptures; they occur most often in patients older than 40 years and in patients with systemic inflammatory diseases such as diabetes and chronic renal disease. With both types of tendon ruptures, the defect resulting from the torn tendon is typically palpable on examination. Patients will also often have significant swelling around the knee. They are unable to actively straighten their leg and will have difficulty with stairs. Surgery is indicated to repair the tendon in patients with an absent extensor mechanism (Figure 5-12) and involves reinsertion of the tendon edges into the bone.

Stress fractures are common overuse injuries seen in athletes due to increased repetitive loading. These fractures are often seen in endurance athletes such as long-distance runners and military personnel. Common locations for these fractures include the tibia, tarsal navicular, metatarsal, and femur (Figure 5-13).[9(pp160-161)] In addition to increased stress on the bone, other risk factors include low estrogen levels in females, poor nutrition, and usage of corticosteroids and NSAIDs. As such, these injuries are often associated with the female athlete triad defined as amenorrhea, eating disorder, and osteoporosis. Initial treatment for these fractures includes activity modification. If symptoms persist, protected weight bearing and use of a bone stimulator can be considered. Under certain conditions, surgery may be necessary for these injuries. For example, if tibial shaft stress fractures involve the anterior cortex, intramedullary nailing should be considered because these fractures have a high likelihood of nonunion. In addition, stress fractures of the femoral neck require surgical fixation if they are tension-side fractures (superior lateral neck) or compression-side fractures (inferior medial neck) involving >50% of the width of the femoral neck.

IV. FRACTURE PATIENTS

Trauma is the fourth leading cause of death in the United States and is the leading cause of death for adults younger than 44 years. Moreover, over half of all trauma patients have orthopaedic injuries.[10] Orthopaedic trauma focuses on fracture care. The treatment of these patients begins at the time of initial evaluation, most often

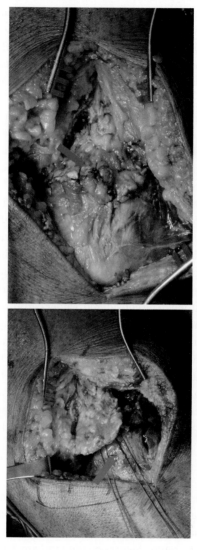

Figure 5-12 Intraoperative images demonstrating suture repair of disrupted quadriceps tendon. Blue arrow points to the patella and red arrow points to where the tendon is reinserted into the superior pole of the patella.

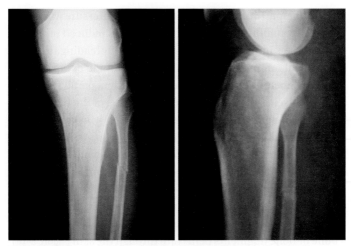

Figure 5-13 Stress fracture. Anteroposterior and lateral radiograph of proximal tibia/fibula demonstrating stress fracture of fibula.

in an emergency room/acute care setting, and continues through the completion of the healing process. These physicians take care of fractures of all areas of the body, some of which involve significant soft tissue and neurovascular damage.

In the trauma bay, orthopaedic injuries are sometimes discovered after a patient has been stabilized from a hemodynamic standpoint and practitioners conduct secondary and tertiary surveys. Any fracture that is recognized should be reduced and immobilized, followed by definitive management as necessary. For some fractures, stabilization can be achieved via splinting and casting; other fractures need surgical intervention and eventual internal fixation. There is a wide range of risks and complications due to traumatic fractures and dislocations, including vascular injury, compartment syndrome, nerve injury, deep vein thrombosis, infection, swelling, and post-traumatic arthritis.

Although many fractures can wait to be definitively fixed, there are three situations that are considered orthopaedic surgical emergencies/urgencies. The first is compartment syndrome, which occurs when there is excessive increased pressure within a muscle compartment (Figure 5-14). Increased pressure within the fascia surrounding the muscle groups causes reduced perfusion to the tissues in that compartment ultimately leading to necrosis. Clinical findings in patients with developing compartment syndrome include pain, paresthesia, palpation, paralysis, pallor, and/or pulselessness (the five "Ps"). Pressure of the tissue compartment of concern can be measured directly using a Stryker pressure monitor device or an arterial line setup. Acute compartment syndrome occurs most often with long bone fractures of the lower leg or the forearm, particularly comminuted fractures. Treatment of impending compartment syndrome involves surgical release of all involved compartments with fasciotomy. The second orthopaedic urgency is an open fracture, fractures where a bone or bone fragments penetrate through the skin (Figure 5-15). Given the risk of infection, these fractures should be debrided and stabilized in the operating room as soon as possible. The

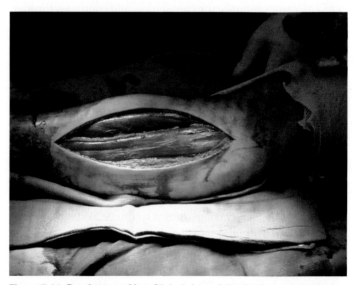

Figure 5-14 Fasciotomy of leg. Clinical picture following four compartment fasciotomy of leg.

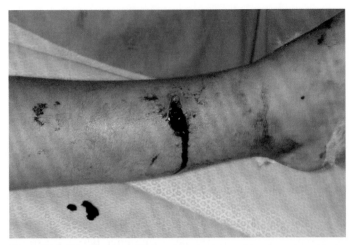

Figure 5-15 **Open fracture.** 18-year-old male status post motorcycle accident with open distal third tibial shaft fracture.

third surgical urgency situation consists of fractures that involve neurologic/vascular injury. Although all fractures are at risk of damaging important neurovascular structures, if a patient presents any sign of neurovascular injury involving delayed capillary refill, weak or absent pulses, or change in sensation, they should be managed acutely to prevent permanent damage.

V. BACK AND SPINE CONDITIONS

Back pain, particularly lower back pain, is one of the more common reasons a patient will visit a doctor's office. Causes of lower back pain include back strain, lumbar disc herniation, and spinal stenosis. Patients suffering from back strain have pain that is localized to the back and buttock region with no radiating pain down the legs. This pain sometime results from a specific trauma or injury; however, the inciting cause is often not known. Symptoms are often exacerbated by bending down or by lifting heavy objects. These patients do not require surgical intervention; they can be treated conservatively with NSAIDs and physical therapy, with most patients' symptoms resolving within 2 weeks. In contrast, patients with herniated lumbar discs (herniated nucleus pulposus, HNP) will complain of radiating pain to the extremities. They will experience pain when bending and/or sitting. On physical examination, tension signs are suggestive of herniated disc pathology. The two discs most commonly involved in lumbar spine disc herniations are the L4-L5 disc and L5-S1 disc (Figure 5-16). Although the cause of this pain is more serious than back strain, these patients also usually do not require surgical intervention. The majority improve with conservative management; discectomy will only be required in about 20% of the cases.

In contrast to patients with HNP, patients suffering lower back pain from spinal stenosis experience pain with spinal

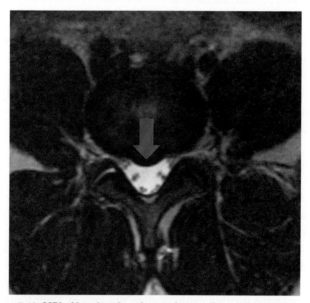

Figure 5-16 MRI of herniated nucleus pulposus. T2-weighted MRI demonstrating a central herniation affecting the lumbar spine. Red arrow demonstrates the herniated disc material.

extension. Patients with spinal stenosis classically complain of referred buttock pain and claudication that is relieved with flexion.[11,12] This condition is characterized by narrowing of the spinal canal or neural foramina causing nerve root compression (Figure 5-17). It is the compression and resultant ischemia that cause pain. If conservative treatment fails, these patients have shown significant improvement with surgical decompression and laminectomy.

Another common complaint related to the spine is neck pain. As with lower back pain, the majority of such complaints are attributed to cervical strain often caused by overuse, stress, poor posture, or sleep positioning. Symptoms of pain and stiffness typically resolve within 6 weeks and may benefit from NSAIDs and physical therapy. Another cause of neck pain is degeneration of

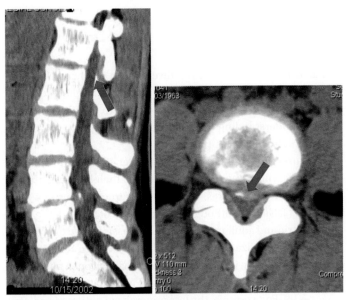

Figure 5-17 CT demonstrating spinal stenosis. Sagittal and axial CT cuts demonstrating spinal stenosis secondary to facet and ligamentum flavum hypertrophy. Arrow demarcates stenosis at L2.

the cervical spine, known as cervical spondylosis. This degeneration, which is part of the natural aging process, can later result in discogenic neck pain, cervical radiculopathy, and cervical myelopathy. Although cervical spondylosis can be the result of age-related wear and tear, when it produces sensory or motor functional impairment, surgical interventions may be desired. Symptoms of cervical myelopathy typically begin with neck pain and stiffness often associated with occipital headaches. Patients can also develop numbness and tingling in their extremities in addition to weakness and clumsiness. They may note that they are dropping objects more frequently or are experiencing difficulty with fine motor skills. Severe disease is characterized by gait instability and difficulty walking up and down stairs. Physical examination in patients with myelopathy is notable for muscle weakness, proprioception deficits, and upper motor neuron signs such as spasticity and hyperreflexia.

VI. PEDIATRIC CONDITIONS

Pediatric orthopaedic care is a diverse field involving the treatment of traumatic, developmental, and congenital orthopaedic injuries in children. Providing proper care to pediatric patients requires understanding the growth and development of children and interacting with their parents.

Fractures are common in children: over 40% of boys and over 25% of girls will sustain a fracture between their birth and the age of 16.[13] Of these fractures, distal forearm fractures are the most common (Table 5-4). Although the principles of care are the same for pediatric and adult patients, with emphasis placed on immobilization and stabilization, it is essential to recognize and factor the differences between immature skeletons (with an open physis) and mature skeletons when one is engaged in pediatric fracture care (Figure 5-18). For example, the less mineralized nature of pediatric bone makes incomplete fractures more common in children. In addition, given the different mechanical properties of pediatric

TABLE 5-4	Frequency of Pediatric Fractures[20]
Fracture Type	**Percentage (%)**
Distal forearm	26
Clavicle	11
Fingers	10
Ankle	7
Toes	5
Metatarsals	5
Distal humerus	5
Metacarpals	5
Facial skeleton	3
Tibia/fibular shaft	3
Proximal forearm	3
Forearm shaft	3
Proximal humerus	3
Carpals	2
Proximal tibia/fibula	1
Ribs	1
Femoral shaft	1
Thoracolumbar spine	1
Distal femur	1
Tarsals	1
Humeral shaft	1
Skull	1
Other sites	1

bone, fractures produce patterns that are unique to children, such as plastic deformation, greenstick fractures, and buckle fractures. Moreover, a child's immature skeleton has a greater capacity to remodel than a mature skeleton. As such, many pediatric fractures

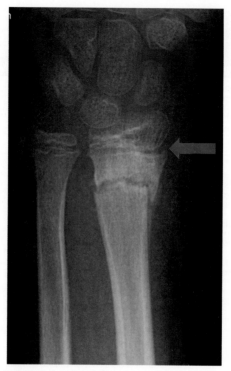

Figure 5-18 **Open physis.** Anteroposterior radiograph of right wrist demonstrating distal radius fracture in a skeletally immature patient. Arrow points to open physis.

may be treated with closed reduction and casting; however, some fractures do require surgical intervention. Fractures that almost always require surgery include fractures that extend into a joint or displace a growth plate, open fractures, elbow fractures, and hip/pelvis/femur fractures (Figure 5-19).[14,15]

Developmental orthopaedic conditions comprise much of the practice of pediatric orthopaedics, with spine and limb deformities being the most common causes of referral. Scoliosis, a coronal or frontal plane curvature of the spine greater than 10 degrees, may lead to severe deformity and even internal organ damage if the

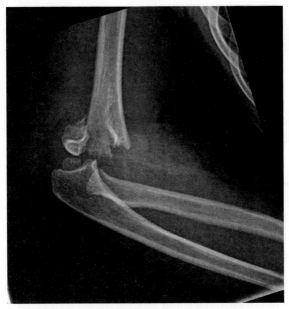

Figure 5-19 Type 3 supracondylar fracture. Lateral radiograph of the elbow demonstrating Type 3 supracondylar fracture. This injury requires reduction and pinning.

degree of curvature becomes severe. Scoliosis is idiopathic in about 80% of cases, but may also be a sign of other conditions including neuromuscular diseases and congenital spine deformities.

DDH is the most common orthopaedic disorder in newborns, occurring in 2 to 5 infants per 1,000.[15] DDH results from abnormal development of the acetabulum causing subluxation and sometimes dislocation of the hip. It is important to detect this condition during newborn screening examinations and correct it with the use of a harness or brace (Figure 5-20). Left untreated, patients will develop further dysplasia of the acetabulum and contraction of the hip muscles, and later treatment is more complicated and less predictable. Other limb disorders include proximal femoral focal deficiency, Legg–Calvé–Perthes disease, and slipped capital femoral epiphysis. Proximal femoral focal deficiency is a congenital

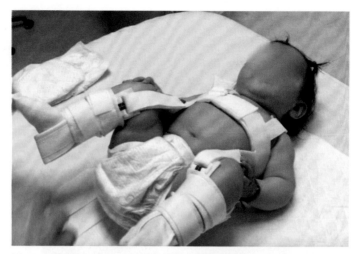

Figure 5-20 Developmental dysplasia of hip (DDH) and harness. Image demonstrating Pavlik harness use in patient with DDH.

defect of the proximal femur ranging from a completely absent hip to a shortened femur. This disorder resulting from a defect in the primary ossification center usually affects one limb causing severe shortening of one leg and resultant leg length discrepancy (Figure 5-21). Several procedures are performed to help these children ambulate. If a patient has a femoral head and the total leg length discrepancy is <20 cm, a leg lengthening procedure may be performed. If there is no femoral head and a severe leg length discrepancy, amputation and ambulation with a prosthesis may be preferred. Legg–Calvé–Perthes disease results from idiopathic avascular necrosis of the proximal femoral epiphysis. Symptoms classically include a painless limp with intermittent hip, knee, or thigh pain. On physical examination, patients will have hip stiffness with little internal rotation and a Trendelenburg gait. Younger patients tend to have better outcomes because the dead bone has time to remodel. Older patients (>8 years old) often require femoral or pelvic osteotomies. Slipped capital femoral epiphysis is a disorder of the proximal femoral physis which results in slipping of

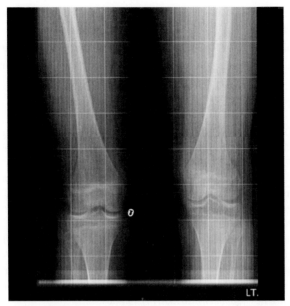

Figure 5-21 Leg length discrepancy. Anteroposterior bilateral femur radiographs demonstrating leg length discrepancy as diagnosed on standing radiographs.

the epiphysis. This is the most common hip disorder in adolescents and is typically seen in obese African American male children. Patients often present with thigh and groin pain in addition to an abnormal gait. Treatment of slipped capital femoral epiphysis is operative in the form of percutaneous cannulated screw fixation.

Congenital disorders in pediatric patient are also commonly seen. These patients often have both orthopaedic and nonorthopaedic conditions. As such, these patients are best treated with the assistance of a care team that understands their unique needs. One such group of disorders is skeletal dysplasia in which the development of bones and cartilage in utero is affected resulting in a variety of anomalies. One of the more common dysplasias is achondroplasia, which is characterized by shortened limbs and an enlarged head. These patients can suffer from many complications, particularly craniocervical junction compression, spinal stenosis, and sleep apnea. These patients often require surgery for their spinal abnormalities including spinal kyphosis and lumbar stenosis and for their genu varum in the form of tibial osteotomies.

REFERENCES

1. Dawson J, Linsell L, Zondervan K, et al. Epidemiology of hip and knee pain and its impact on overall health status in older adults. *Rheumatology*. 2004;43(4):497-504.
2. Zhang W, Moskowitz RW, Nuki G, et al. OARSI recommendations for the management of hip and knee osteoarthritis. Part II: OARSI evidence-based, expert consensus guidelines. *Osteoarthr Cartil*. 2008;16:137-162.
3. Jevsevar D. Treatment of osteoarthritis of the knee: evidence-based guideline, 2nd Edition. *J Am Acad Orthop Surg*. 2013;21:571-576.
4. Moyer RF, Birimgham TB, Bryant DM, et al. Valgus bracing for knee osteoarthritis: a meta-analysis of randomized trials. *Arthritis Care Res (Hoboken)*. 2015;67(4):493-501.
5. Bellamy N, Campbell J, Robinson V, Gee T, Bourne R, Wells G. Intraarticular corticosteroid for treatment of osteoarthritis of the knee. *Cochrane Database Syst Rev*. 2006;(2):CD005328.
6. HCPUnet, Healthcare Cost and Utilization Project. Agency for Healthcare Research and Quality. http://hcupnet.ahrq.gov. Accessed August 8, 2016.
7. Berry DJ, von Knoch M, Schleck CD, Harmsen WS. The cumulative long-term risk of dislocation after primary Charnley total hip arthroplasty. *J Bone Joint Surg Am*. 2004;86-A(1):9-14.
8. Gelfman R, Melton LJ, Yawn BP, Wollan PC, Amadio PC, Stevens JC. Long-term trends in carpal tunnel syndrome. *Neurology*. 2009;72(1):33-41.
9. Maak TG, Rodeo SA. *DeLee and Drez's Orthopaedic Sports Medicine*. 4th ed. Philadelphia, PA: Saunders; 2015:1117.
10. Centers for Disease Control and Prevention. WISQARS, injury prevention & control: data and statistics. http://www.cdc.gov/injury/wisqars/index.html. Accessed August 8, 2016.
11. Katz JN, Harris MD. Clinical practice. Lumbar spinal stenosis. *N Engl J Med*. 2008;358(8):818.

12. Hall S, Bartleson JD, Onofrio BM. Lumbar spinal stenosis. Clinical features, diagnostic procedures, and results of surgical treatment in 68 patients. *Ann Intern Med.* 1985;103(2):271.

13. Landin LA. Epidemiology of children's fractures. *J Pediatr Orthop B.* 1997;6:79-83.

14. Wiesel BB, Sankar WN, Delahay JN, Wiesel SW. O*rthopedic Surgery: Principles of Diagnosis and Treatment.* Philadelphia, PA: Wolters Kluwer Health/Lippincott Williams & Wilkins, 2011;401.

15. Canale ST, Beaty JH. *Campbell's Operative Orthopaedics* 12th ed. Philadelphia, PA: Mosby, 2013;1365.

16. Bialik V, Bialik GM, Blazer S, Sujov P, Wiener F, Berant M. Developmental dysplasia of the hip: a new approach to incidence. *Pediatrics.* 1999;103(1):93-99.

17. Moss AS, Murphy LB, Helmick CG, Schwartz TA, Barbour KE, Renner JB, et al. Annual incidence rates of hip symptoms and three hip OA outcomes from a U.S. population-based cohort study: the Johnston County Osteoarthritis Project. *Osteoarthr Cartil.* 2016; 24(9):1518-1527.

18. Murphy LB, Moss S, Do BT, Helmick CG, Schwartz TA, Barbour KE, et al. Annual incidence of knee symptoms and four knee osteoarthritis outcomes in the Johnston Country Osteoarthritis Project. *Arthritis Care Res (Hoboken).* 2016;68(1):55-65.

19. Chung KC, Spilson SV. The frequency and epidemiology of hand and forearm fractures in the United States. *J Hand Surg Am.* 2001;26(5):908-915.

20. Hedstrom EM, Svensson O, Bergstrom U, Michno P. Epidemiology of fractures in children and adolescents. *Acta Orthop.* 2010;81(1):148-153.

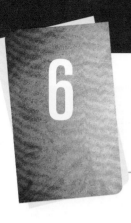

6

OPERATIVE MANAGEMENT

Avraham Schulgasser

I. GOALS OF SURGERY AND OUTCOME EXPECTATIONS

There are numerous reasons to perform orthopaedic surgery which are usually categorized as elective or nonelective cases. Elective cases are nonemergent and for the most part aim at improving quality of life in one way or the other. Nonelective cases are generally urgent or emergent, but also serve to improve quality of life while possibly preventing or delaying further progression of injury or disease process. The primary goals of surgery are: restoration of anatomic parameter status postinjury, infection control, pain relief, return to baseline functional level, and prevention of further damage.[1]

Restoration of proper anatomic parameters encompasses a variety of cases such as fracture repair and repair of congenital or acquired malformation. In cases of a displaced fracture, surgery is beneficial, in that once fracture reduction and limb alignment are restored functional recovery generally follows. A fracture that heals incorrectly can drastically reduce range of motion to the affected limb or joint, limiting the ability to perform ADLs. By restoring anatomic parameters, surgery may often help prevent or delay the onset of posttraumatic arthritis that may occur with fractures involving joints (intra-articular).[2] For congenital abnormalities, surgical correction may help reduce or eliminate some of the long-term complications that once, years ago, might have been irreparable.

In the case of open wounds (Figure 6-1) or in the setting of established musculoskeletal infection, surgical debridement is needed to reduce the incidence or treat the cause of contamination. This

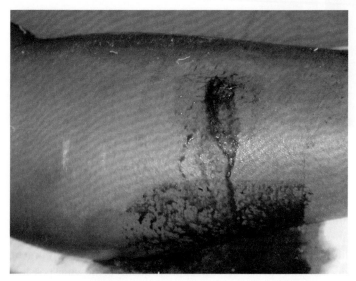

Figure 6-1 **Open wound.** An open wound requiring surgical debridement.

includes irrigation and debridement of open wounds and septic joints or removal of hardware or implants when infection is present. In some cases, it is essential to remove the affected hardware because oral and intravenous antibiotics cannot penetrate foreign bodies to eliminate an infection. Multiple surgeries may be required depending on the situation. Once the infection clears, revision prostheses or hardware may be needed in order to fix the fracture or joint.

Pain relief is probably the most common indicator for surgery. A prime example of this is total joint arthroplasty. Patients with debilitating arthritis can get significant relief with joint replacement surgery. Additionally, in cases where patients previously underwent surgery to repair a fracture and now have discomfort from the implanted hardware, a removal of hardware may provide much needed pain relief. Additional situations in which pain relief is the primary goal include discectomy and spinal fusion for back and lower extremity pain and neurolysis for neuropathic pain syndromes.

Another indication for orthopaedic surgical intervention is prevention or delay of further injury progression. Some cases include unstable fracture patterns that without fixation will ultimately heal in malunion.[3] Carpal tunnel/cubital tunnel release surgery works to prevent progression of nerve injury, and tumor removal to prevent further spread of cancerous lesions.[4]

Patient expectations can vary depending on the nature of the need for surgery whether it be restorative, to control infection, for pain relief, or to inhibit progression. More complex injuries may have a less favorable outcome than simpler ones. Patients with advanced stages of arthritis will have a longer road to recovery than those with earlier stages. This may be due to inactivity of patients with advanced arthritis, which can lead to muscle atrophy. Additionally, in patients who develop contractures, it can take longer to regain mobility. It is important that the patient is aware of all of the relevant variables to prevent false expectations.[5] As with all surgeries, there are inherent risks that patients must be made aware of. Although great lengths are taken to minimize all risks, disclosure and transparency are important, and patients must be informed of possible negative consequences.

The goal of all surgery is to have the patient ultimately emerge in a better state of health than prior to surgery. Many variables factor in, and these will play a large part in individual outcomes.

Timeline and Progression of Healing

The timeline and progression of healing vary greatly depending on the procedure performed and the condition of the patient preoperatively and postoperatively. Age, physical condition, emotional stability, and patient cooperation and compliance all play a part in the healing process. Patients who undergo simple joint replacements such as hips and knees might expect to be weight bearing within the first day or two after surgery. However, patients who undergo a tendon repair typically require weeks of immobilization followed by extensive physical or occupational therapy to allow for proper healing. Simpler procedures such as trigger finger and carpal tunnel release only require a few weeks of recovery and often do not need any type of therapy. Fractures, depending on location and severity of the injury, will also vary in the length of time it takes before full healing is achieved. Just as patients must be apprised of the risks inherent in their specific surgery, so too should they be apprised of the realistic timeline range and successive recovery stages that they might expect.

II. CLEARANCE AND PREOPERATIVE TESTING

As with all patients, a thorough history is an essential component of the patient examination. In the surgical patient, this is especially critical to ensure that all appropriate measures are taken prior to surgery. A thorough history and knowledge of preexisting medical conditions allow for the optimization of the patient prior to surgery and limit possible complications caused by unanticipated variables. Detailed history of prior anesthesia complications, as well as cardiac, pulmonary, endocrinology, and other pertinent medical comorbidities is essential.[6]

In emergent cases, preoperative clearances may be expedited and obtained by in-house medical providers. For elective cases, patients have more time and could typically be seen by their own health care providers. This of course will typically take more time to arrange and coordinate.

Depending on the patient, a specific set of preoperative tests are required (Table 6-1). Local policies and procedures as well as sound clinical judgment should be used on an individual patient-by-patient basis.

III. PREOPERATIVE CONSIDERATIONS AND INSTRUCTIONS

Skin Preparation

It is crucial to do a thorough skin examination of the area prior to surgery. It is important to note any prior surgical incisions or lesions that may fall in the path of the usual incision site. Sometimes

6-1 Suggested Preoperative Testing Guidelines Based on Demographics and Comorbidities

	Suggested Preoperative Testing Guidelines								
	Medical Evaluation	CBC	UA	Coags	BMP	Hepatic Panel	CXR	EKG	Other
Age and Sex									
Neonates–6 mo		X							
Menarche–menopause		X							Urine pregnancy
50 and over		X						X	
65 and over	X	X			X			X	
Medical Condition									
Cardiovascular and cerebrovascular disease	X	X			X			X	
Pulmonary disease	X	X			X		X	X	
Sleep apnea	X	X			X			X	
Diabetes	X	X			X			X	HgbA1c
Hepatic disease	X	X		X	X	X		X	
Renal disease	X	X	X		X			X	
Bleeding disorder	X	X		X					Type and screen
BMI >40	X	X			X	X		X	
Malignancy on chemo	X	X			X	X		X	
HTN	X				X			X	
Neuromuscular disease, seizures	X								
Alcohol abuse				X	X	X			
Hx anemia	X	X							

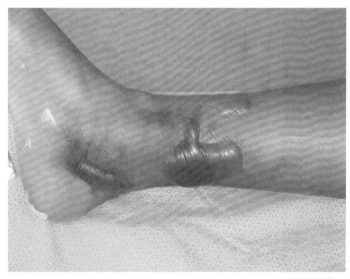

Figure 6-2 **Fracture blisters.** Fracture blisters as evidenced by the fluid-filled vesicles and bullae overlying the fracture site.

in the trauma patient, surgery will need to be delayed to allow for swelling to diminish and fracture blisters to heal prior to operating on a patient (Figure 6-2). This delay helps reduce possible wound complications.[7] In elective cases where there is a preexisting skin condition, patients would be better served with a short course of treatment prior to surgery to help diminish any possibility of wound complications. Additionally, patients should be instructed to elevate and ice limbs whenever possible prior to surgery, specifically in trauma cases.

In complicated cases where incisions involve areas of previous skin grafting, severe swelling, complex lacerations in the surgical field, areas where cosmesis is of concern, or general concerns regarding wound healing, a plastic surgeon should be consulted for further evaluation. Depending on the complexity, plastic surgeons may need to assist with the incision and closure of the surgical wound.

NPO

As part of the preoperative instructions patients should be advised to remain NPO prior to surgery. Typically, this means from midnight prior to surgery. In cases where surgery must be performed emergently or is scheduled for later in the day, refer to local policies and procedures in regard to NPO status.

Medications

As stated earlier, it is essential to gather a thorough history and make note of all medications the patient is currently taking. This includes over-the-counter, prescribed, or other available supplements a patient may be on. Many medications may be safely continued up to and throughout the perioperative period while some medications may need to be held. Some of the following cardiac medications can be continued as prescribed even on the day of surgery: beta-blockers, calcium channel blockers, ACE inhibitors, and statins. Diuretics should be held on the morning of surgery. Oral contraceptives when possible should be stopped a few weeks prior to surgery to prevent DVT. However, careful consideration must be taken to ensure the prevention of unwanted pregnancy. Another population encountered is diabetics. They can typically continue with oral antiglycemic agents until the morning of surgery. For those on insulin, dosing must be adjusted to account for the NPO period and duration of surgery. Patients taking blood thinners will require labs to assess PT/PTT/INR. These medications will need to be held prior to surgery to prevent excess operative blood loss. Typically, anticoagulants are held for a few days prior to elective surgery.[8] Careful history is essential to balance risks versus benefits depending on the patient's history. As a general rule, patients with multiple medical comorbidities on multiple medications should be evaluated by their primary care physician to ensure appropriate management and follow-up. Additionally, patients taking homeopathic medications should be advised to discontinue these medications a few days prior to surgery (Table 6-2).

TABLE 6-2 Commonly Used Herbal Medicines, Their Uses, Effects, and Perioperative Considerations

Herbal Medicine	Uses	Pharmacologic effects	Perioperative considerations	Discontinuation recommendation
Echinacea	Improve immune system	Modulates cytokines; stimulates macrophages and NK cells	Avoid known hepatotoxic drugs	No data available; discontinue 2 wk before surgery
Ephedra	CNS stimulant; weight loss; asthma treatment	Sympathomimetic	Caution with other sympathomimetics; arrhythmias with halothane	Discontinue 24 h before surgery
Garlic	Treatment of hypertension, hyperlipidemia, atherosclerosis	Antiplatelet effects	Risk of bleeding	Discontinue 7 d before surgery
Ginger	Anti-inflammatory; antiemetic	Inhibit serotonergic pathways; stimulate GI tract	Risk of bleeding	No data available. Discontinue 2 wk before surgery

Ginkgo biloba	Neuroprotective; improves blood flow	Free radical scavenger; antiplatelet effects	Risk of bleeding	Discontinue 36 h before surgery
Ginseng	Mood enhancer; aphrodisiac	Sympathomimetic	Risk of bleeding; hypoglycemic effect; caution with other sympathomimetics	Discontinue 7 d before surgery
Kava	Sedative; anxiolytic	Potentiate GABA-mediated system	Reduce anesthetic requirements	Discontinue 24 h before surgery
St John's wort	Antidepressant	Inhibit MAOIs; induces cytochrome p450	Serotonergic crisis; sedative effect	Discontinue 5 d before surgery
Valerian	Anxiolytic; hypnotic	Potentiate GABA-ergic system	Reduce anesthetic requirements	No data available; discontinue 2 wk before surgery

From Wong A, Townley SA. Herbal medicines and anaesthesia. *Contin Educ Anaesth Crit Care Pain.* 2011;11(1):14-17.

Initiation of Postoperative Care Arrangements

Postoperative care arrangements should be made when surgical planning is taking place. It is important to note whether the case will be booked as inpatient or ambulatory. In instances where the surgery will be a same-day procedure it is necessary to ensure that the patient has transportation and a safe location to return to. Elderly patients or those who live alone often require the additional support of their family or friends or of a home health aide. Longer, more complicated surgeries often require that the patient be admitted or sent to a rehabilitation center. Arrangements for rehabilitation should be made in advance whenever possible because many insurances require preauthorizations. With newer bundled care initiatives, there has been a push to discharge patients home instead of rehabilitation. Within the inpatient setting, these matters are usually handled by a case worker or a social worker.[9]

Return to School, Work, Volunteering, Sport, and Driving

The timeline to return to school or work, sports, and driving will again vary depending on the type of procedure performed. At the very minimum, it is generally recommended that patients plan on taking at least 1 week for recovery.

Patients' return to work depends on their occupation. In instances where patients have desk-type responsibilities rather than duties that are physically demanding, they may return to work sooner. The decision to return to work must take into consideration the patient's ability to commute to where they need to go. Whether the patient drives, is driven, or takes public transportation are all variables for consideration.

IV. WHAT TO EXPECT ON THE DAY OF SURGERY

Arrival Time for Staff and Patients

For staff, the time to arrive prior to surgery will vary based on the type of practice and its location. As a good rule of thumb, those involved in the surgery should plan to arrive at least 45 to 60 minutes prior to the first scheduled surgery of the day. This will allow time to review the cases and make certain of familiarity with the specifics and all relevant details. It also allows time to meet with and brief the surgical team. This helps ensure that the procedure runs smoothly and that all facets of the surgery are accounted for.

For the patient, arrival time will depend on the necessary paperwork, the procedure, and whether the setting is impatient or outpatient. In some cases, the patient will be admitted to the facility prior to the scheduled surgery. Inpatient admission prior to surgery allows for close monitoring and optimization of the acute patient. The majority of these cases will be trauma patients admitted through the emergency department. In instances of ambulatory surgery or procedures performed in surgical centers, patients may arrive at least an hour prior to their scheduled procedure.

Expectations for Discharge

A common concern of patients is in regard to when they will be discharged after surgery. There has been an increasing popularity for same-day discharges; however, this will be determined based on a number of factors. For simpler procedures in which the patient is stable after surgery, the patient can be discharged same day. Typically, patients will need to remain in recovery for a few hours to allow for anesthesia to wear off and for routine monitoring. Additionally, in many facilities, patients may receive rapid rehabilitation by trained therapists for mobilization and other services prior to their discharge to ensure that they will be safe once they leave. Upon discharge, patients should be instructed on proper medication dosing (ie, pain medications, antibiotics, DVT prophylaxis, etc.), wound/bandage care, signs to look out for that may indicate complications, and when to follow-up in the outpatient office/clinic.

With more complex and lengthy procedures, patients should expect to be admitted to the hospital for an overnight or longer stay. Indications for admission include: extended operating time, infection, intraoperative blood loss, anesthesia complications, and procedures complicated by the management of multiple medical comorbidities. Additionally, patients who have no safe place to return to after surgery may need to be admitted until appropriate arrangements can be made.

Length of Surgery and General Plan

The length of surgery will depend on the procedure being performed and the skill of the provider. Simple cases such as trigger finger and carpal tunnel releases take just a few minutes. Often the setup and anesthesia take longer than the actual case. More complicated spine cases or reconstructive surgeries can last quite a few hours. It is important to be familiar with the procedures performed in your practice on a routine basis so that patients can be educated and can be given realistic expectations.

Anesthesia

There are a variety of options in regard to anesthesia available. They can be divided into general, regional, and local. Under general anesthesia, patients are completely unconscious and have no sensations. These patients may need to be intubated or at least have a laryngeal mask airway to ensure that airway is maintained and require the closest monitoring. This type of anesthesia is preferable for lengthy procedures and where complete paralysis is beneficial. Instances where paralysis is beneficial include cases where traction is needed for proper fracture reduction.

With neuraxial (spinal) and peripheral nerve blocks patients can remain alert if they choose, because these anesthetics have a localized effect on pain sensation. Neuraxial blocks provide greater coverage because they work on the nerve at the level of the spinal cord, whereas peripheral blocks allow us to target a smaller region. Oftentimes, more than one regional block will be administered because the coverage areas overlap, allowing for better pain control. In addition to the block, these patients will receive a sedative to help them sleep and diminish memory of the procedure. Depending on the medication administered, the duration of the block will vary. See Table 6-3 for commonly used regional nerve blocks.

TABLE 6-3	Commonly Used Peripheral Nerve Blocks
Block Type	**Coverage Area**
Interscalene	Procedures from shoulder to midshaft humerus
Supraclavicular	Procedures from midshaft humerus to hand
Infraclavicular	Procedures distal to the elbow
Axillary	Procedures of the forearm and hand
Forearm (radial, ulnar, median)	Procedures of the hand and wrist
Wrist (radial, ulnar, median)	Procedures of the hand and finger
Femoral	Anterior thigh, femur, knee
Saphenous	Supplementation for medial foot/ankle surgery in combination with a sciatic nerve block
Sciatic	Foot and ankle surgery
Popliteal	Foot and ankle surgery

From Hadzic A. *Hadzic's Peripheral Nerve Blocks and Anatomy for Ultrasound-Guided Regional Anesthesia*. 2nd ed. New York, NY: McGraw-Hill; 2012.

Lastly, patients may receive local blocks. As the name indicates, these are more superficial and localized to small regions. They are preferred for more superficial procedures and are of limited use in larger procedures. They are often injected at incision site to help diminish postoperative pain or for simple procedures such as laceration repair.

Postoperative Pain Management

An important aspect of postsurgical care is adequate pain management. When considering various analgesics, it is important to find out from the patient if there are any drug allergies, if they are on chronic pain management, or if they have other medical comorbidities that will affect dosing.

In our practice, whenever possible, we have our patients receive preoperative peripheral nerve blocks. This helps minimize the initial postoperative pain. These blocks can last up to 12 to 24 hours. However, this will vary based on the particular medication injected. The drawback to regional blocks is that many patients will experience a rebound pain as the block wears off. Patients should be advised of this and instructed to begin taking oral analgesics prior to the block wearing off, to allow for continuous pain control.[10] In addition to nerve blocks patients are often injected with local analgesics at the surgical site. Newer local agents can have an effect for up to 3 days.[11] However, these are mainly used after joint replacement, owing to the cost-prohibitive nature of the medication. They will likely be used more universally once their efficacy can be demonstrated in place of initial narcotic use. In the inpatient setting, postoperative patients are often treated with IV analgesics or patient-controlled anesthesia (PCA). With PCA pumps, patients are afforded the ability to control to some degree how much and how often they receive IV analgesics. Dose limits are preset by the ordering provider to ensure that the patient can only receive a safe dose.

Most patients are sent home with oral analgesics such as opioid-based narcotics. Patients should be instructed on maximal daily doses and advised to wean off these medications as soon as possible. Special consideration must be taken for the elderly and patients who are chronic drug users. Often, patients in our practice will be referred to pain management specialists if there is a concern for abuse.

When managing the pain of postoperative fracture patients, NSAIDs can be used as adjuvant therapy to minimize immediate postoperative pain. There is some concern that NSAIDs may delay fracture healing, but the literature is unclear.[12] For patients where this is not a concern, NSAIDs can effectively be used along opioid narcotics to prevent breakthrough pain and extend the interval between narcotic doses.

In addition to medication we instruct all our patients to keep the operated limb elevated and iced whenever possible to help minimize swelling. A common cause of discomfort is extensive swelling at the surgical site. For patients who are splinted with excessive pain, the splint can be loosened, which often yields significant pain relief.

Weight-Bearing Status and Restrictions

Weight-bearing status will depend on the procedure performed and individual provider preferences. In the case of simple joint replacement, patients are weight bearing immediately postsurgery. In instances where this is complicated by fracture, patients may be only partial weight bearing until there is further healing of the fracture. Many lower extremity articular fractures such as calcaneal and tibial plateau fractures will require the patient be nonweight bearing for up to 2 to 3 months. Rotational ankle fractures can typically begin being weight bearing after 6 weeks.

In addition to weight-bearing status, patients may be restricted on extent of range of motion. Even in cases where patients are made weight bearing immediately postoperatively, there may be limitations on impact activities.

V. POSTOPERATIVE FOLLOW-UP FOR THE OUTPATIENT

Postoperative Day 1 Contact

With the increased push for same-day ambulatory procedures, it is imperative to maintain close follow-up on the postoperative patient. Too often patients are discharged without receiving adequate postoperative instructions or upon their return home find that they have additional questions that they did not think about or simply forgot to ask. It is always a good idea to contact all discharged patients on postoperative day 1. This allows you to address any concerns that may have come up. It also allows the care team to review and clarify postoperative instructions such as proper medication dosages, ensuring DVT prophylaxis compliance when warranted, bandage and wound care, as well as procedure-specific instructions. We also use this time to remind our patients when they need to return for follow-up and when to seek emergency care. It is a simple but effective way to ensure patients do not get lost to follow-up and an important role that the Advanced Practice Provider plays in the practice.

Initial Postoperative Visit

In many practices, the initial postoperative visit serves a number of key purposes. It serves as a forum to address any concerns and questions that the patient may still have. It allows us to assess the wound healing and when necessary remove any sutures or staples. In many arthroplasty practices, the immediate care such as suture removal is provided by visiting nurse services or at a rehab center. Pain level is assessed as well and any necessary changes to pain regimen can be made. Depending on the practice protocol and procedure performed, new imaging may be obtained at this visit as well to ensure implants are in proper position and joints are still well reduced. Often patients will be transitioned from more cumbersome splints to more comfortable braces or casts if needed. In many cases, during this appointment we will initiate outpatient physical therapy and referral to any other required services such as pain management, infectious disease, etc. Often patients will bring in work or insurance documentation that will need to be completed postsurgery.

Subsequent Postoperative Visits

The subsequent postoperative visits allow you to follow your patient's progress and address any new issues or concerns along the way. These appointments usually follow some protocol, which varies by provider. There are many times when the regular intervals change depending on the need for closer or less frequent observation. In instances of fracture repair, these visits allow us to review new imaging and ensure that healing is progressing as expected. In other instances, close follow-up may be necessary to ensure infection is under control or patients are progressing with functional goals such as joint range of motion and strength. Additionally, these visits allow you to modify physical therapy regimens as needed. Neurovascular status and pain control are also assessed.

Imaging Expectations

What imaging and when imaging is obtained will vary based on the procedure performed and by the individual provider. Plain radiography is still the mainstay of all orthopaedic practice because these films still proved a safe and effective method for initial musculoskeletal evaluation. In fracture management, X-rays are relied on heavily to ensure that the fracture is healing properly. With each subsequent X-ray we expect to see further consolidation of the fracture. Plain films are also relied on heavily after joint replacement surgery. These X-rays allow us to ensure that the joint is well reduced and screen for implant complications such as polyethylene wear or signs of implant loosening. Oftentimes, plain films alone do not provide enough information. Such cases include instances where we need confirmation or are unsure of fracture union. Under these circumstances, a CT scan is a useful test. CT scans are essential in that they compile multiple X-ray slices and provide a three-dimensional image which allows us to get a full sense of bone healing or lack thereof. Additionally, MRI can be used to assess for avascular necrosis or associated soft-tissue injury. In general, MRI is relied on heavily to assess soft-tissue injuries such as ligamentous sprains, muscle tears, cartilage wear, etc., because plain films do not allow us to properly assess these soft-tissue injuries. Nuclear imaging such as labeled bone scans can also be obtained to help determine whether there is a mass of infection, fracture union, or metastatic tumor.

Newer imaging technology is constantly on the horizon. One such technology is EOS imaging. This system produces high-resolution 3D X-ray images and uses significantly less radiation than standard plain films or CT scan. It is currently used for obtaining standing images in the pediatric population to evaluate the spine.

Discharge and Maximal Medical Improvement

Discharge to follow-up as needed varies on the procedure performed. In the case of a total joint replacement, for example, patients should continue follow-up every 1 or 2 years to assess implant position and wear. With smaller procedures such as trigger finger releases, patients may need to be followed only for a few months. Fracture patients are typically followed for 1 year postsurgery because that is the length of time required for many of these patients to reach their maximal medical improvement (aka MMI). MMI is achieved when there is no longer an expectation for improvement in the patient's condition. This expectation could be due to the fact that patients have fully healed or rather that everything possible surgically and nonsurgically was done and there is no more reasonable expectation for improvement. It is important to recognize when your patient has reached their MMI as disability ratings depend on this MMI. Depending on the injury, the length of time needed to reach MMI will vary. Refer to Chapter 9 for a more detailed discussion along with guidelines to determining whether a patient can be classified as having reached the MMI.

Sequelae

Even in the best managed patients, there are events that are sometimes beyond control. Fractures can fail to unite, infection can occur, and arthroplasty can fail. In the event of a nonunion, it is important to identify the cause. It can be due to a mechanical or biologic process. Mechanical processes include inadequate fixation or undersized implants that allow for movement at the fracture site. Additional cause or mechanical process can include weight bearing before enough healing has taken place. Biologic causes include infection and poor blood supply to fracture site. Additional risk factors for nonunion include smoking, diabetes, and patients with hypothyroidism. When working up patients for suspected nonunion, a CT scan and labs should be acquired. CT scans are invaluable in confirming the diagnosis (Figure 6-3) and lab work to rule out infection.

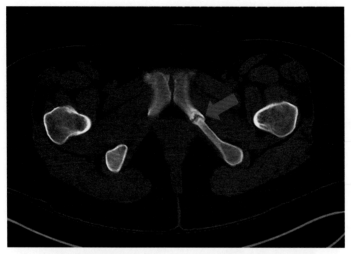

Figure 6-3 CT of nonunion. Axial CT image demonstrating nonunion of the left inferior pubic ramus. Red arrow points to a hypertrophic nonunion of the pubic ramus.

Other sequelae includes infection of the surgical site. In these cases, all hardware may or may not be removed and the infection site thoroughly irrigated and debrided along with the initiation of IV or PO antibiotics.

Periprosthetic fractures (Figure 6-4) are another complication that occasionally arise in postoperative patients. Patients with untreated osteoporosis are at high risk for periprosthetic fractures because of their brittle bone. Age-related osteoporosis is common in postmenopausal females because the decline in estrogen leads to a hormone imbalance in which bone is broken down at a quicker rate than it can be rebuilt. Inadequate intake of calcium and vitamin D also can contribute to weaker bone. Additionally, osteoporosis can be due to iatrogenic causes. One of the most common iatrogenic causes is the use of medications. Glucocorticoid medications as well as a number of common cancer treatment medications are largely responsible for iatrogenic osteoporosis.[13] For these patient demographics, frequent screening and medication management are essential to reduce their risk of fracture.

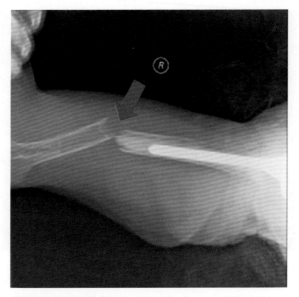

Figure 6-4 Periprosthetic fracture. Lateral radiograph of the right humerus demonstrates a periprosthetic fracture (Red Arrow) below a long stem prosthesis.

Additional sequelae include osteonecrosis, excessive scar tissue formation, or heterotrophic ossification, which may cause discomfort and impede joint range of motion. Nerve injury may also occur at the time of injury or as the result of an iatrogenic injury (Figure 6-5). This can lead to temporary or permanent deficits in sensation and motor function.

VI. POSTOPERATIVE FOLLOW-UP FOR THE INPATIENT

Rounding

Postoperatively, it is essential to round on all inpatients. This ensures patients are receiving proper care while admitted to the hospital. For patients who need the care of additional services, it allows for a review of their recommendations and provides a cohesive plan of care. Additionally, this time is used to address any of the patient's questions or concerns. Often, patients will have family,

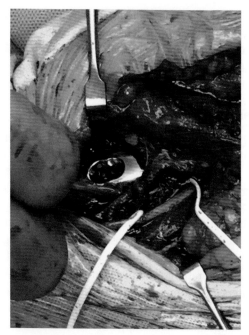

Figure 6-5 **Vessel loop is around the radial nerve during an anterolateral appraoch to the humerus.**

friends, or others who may be caring for them present and this offers time to speak with them and relay important information regarding the patient's care.

Consults to Pain Management, Infectious Disease, and Rehabilitation

While patients are admitted, there is the opportunity to utilize services within the hospital to optimize patients' care. These services may include: Pain Management, Infectious Disease, Medicine, Social Services, and Rehabilitation. Depending on the patient, there may be a need to utilize a few or all of these services. For all patients being followed for infection, the Infectious Disease service should be consulted. Similarly, patients with multiple medical comorbidities should be followed by the Medicine service or hospitalist. In most hospitals, the orthopaedic patient will be evaluated and treated by Physical/Occupational Therapy. Depending on the work location, the available services may vary. One should familiarize oneself with the available resources to ensure the best possible care for patients.

Acute versus Subacute Rehabilitation

For those patients where discharge to home is not appropriate, a rehabilitation center is the best course of action for discharge planning. There are two possible rehabilitation options: acute or subacute. The patient's needs will help determine which is best suited. Acute rehabilitation is generally for a shorter stay than subacute rehabilitation. This is most suitable for patients with multiple medical comorbidities requiring close medical monitoring and daily monitoring by a physician/nonphysician provider and also require daily labs and alterations in course of medical management. Acute rehab centers are better prepared to deal in-house with any complications that may arise. Generally, patients will receive intensive physical and occupational therapy, often in excess of 3 hours daily.[14]

In subacute rehabilitation, therapy usually takes up less time and typical lengths of stay are longer. Patients are not necessarily seen by physicians, PAs, or NPs daily and may be followed by ancillary medical staff. Subacute rehabilitation is best suited for patients who have undergone procedures such as joint replacement or fracture repair who do not have other medical comorbidities and/or do not have ample support to return home safely.

Follow-Up in the Outpatient Setting

Depending on the type of setting and practice protocols, follow-up will vary. We tend to see patients return between 10 and 14 days for wound checks and suture removal, and then in increasing intervals until approximately 1-year postoperation. For patients with joint replacements, continual monitoring is necessary and follow-up is maintained every few years. Practice protocol and provider preference will dictate a follow-up regimen. You will become familiar with your own supervising physician's protocols.

REFERENCES

1. Mackenzie CR, Su EP. Surgical treatment of joint diseases. In: Goldman L, Schafer AI, eds. *Goldman-Cecil Medicine*. 25th ed. Philadelphia, PA: Elsevier/Saunders; 2016:1828-1833.
2. Schenker ML, Mauck RL, Ahn J, Mehta S. Pathogenesis and prevention of posttraumatic osteoarthritis after intra-articular fracture. *J Am Acad Orthop Surg*. 2014;22(1):20-28. doi:10.5435/JAAOS-22-01-20.
3. Leslie MP, Baumgaertner MR. Intertrochanteric hip fractures. In: Browner B, Jupiter J, Krettek C, Anderson P, eds. *Skeletal Trauma: Basic Science, Management, and Reconstruction*. 5th ed. Philadelphia, PA: Saunders; 2015:1683-1720.
4. McNab I, Tucker S. Carpal tunnel syndrome. In: *Disorders of the Hand*. Vol 2. 2015th ed. New York, NY: Springer; 2014:217-229.
5. Witiw CD, Mansouri A, Mathieu F, Nassiri F, Badhiwala JH, Fessler RG. Exploring the expectation-actuality discrepancy: a systematic review of the impact of preoperative expectations on satisfaction and patient reported outcomes in spinal surgery. *Neurosurg Rev*. 2016. doi:10.1007/s10143-016-0720-0
6. Fischer SP. Cost-effective preoperative evaluation and testing. *CHEST J*. 1999;115(suppl 2):96S-100S.
7. Fulkerson EW, Egol KA. Timing issues in fracture management. *Bull NYU Hosp Joint Dis*. 2009;67(1):58-67.
8. Muluk V, Cohn SL, Whinney C. Perioperative medication management. In: Auerbach AD, Holt NF, eds. *UpToDate*. Waltham, MA: UpToDate; 2011.
9. Davidson KW. Evolving social work roles in health care: the case of discharge planning. *Soc Work Health Care*. 1978;4(1):43-54.
10. Goldstein RY, Montero N, Jain SK, Egol KA, Tejwani NC. Efficacy of popliteal block in postoperative pain control after ankle fracture fixation: a prospective randomized study. *J Orthop Trauma*. 2012;26(10):557-561.
11. Portillo J, Kamar N, Melibary S, Quevedo E, Bergese S. Safety of liposome extended-release bupivacaine for postoperative pain control. *Front Pharmacol*. 2014;5:90.
12. Marquez-Lara A, Hutchinson ID, Nuñez F, Smith TL, Miller AN. Nonsteroidal anti-inflammatory drugs and bone-healing. *JBJS Rev*. 2016;4(3):e4.
13. Lindsay R, Cosman F. Osteoporosis. In: Kasper D, Fauci A, Hauser S, Longo D, Jameson J, Loscalzo J. eds. *Harrison's Principles of Internal Medicine*. 19th ed. New York, NY: McGraw-Hill; 2015.
14. Paniagua MA, Bradway C, Eskildsen MA. Chapter 172: Hospital discharge to the nursing home. In: McKean SC, Ross JJ, Dressler DD, Brotman DJ, Ginsberg JS, eds. *Principles and Practice of Hospital Medicine*. New York, NY: McGraw-Hill; 2012.

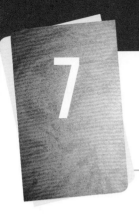

NONOPERATIVE ORTHOPAEDIC CONDITIONS

Rebekah Belayneh and Kenneth A. Egol

I. GOALS OF TREATMENT AND OUTCOME EXPECTATIONS

The majority of musculoskeletal complaints are treated with non-operative therapies. The primary goals of nonoperative management for an orthopaedic patient are to decrease pain, maximize functional outcomes, and restore the patient's ability to perform daily activities of living in a timely manner after treatment. These goals can be accomplished with comprehensive understanding of the entire injury or condition, including fracture, bone deformities, soft-tissue injuries, skin manifestations, swelling, location of pain and/or tenderness, and the overall mechanical demands of the joint involved. Goals of treatment and expected functional and health-related quality of life outcomes can be established with a full appreciation of the injury.[1]

For a nonoperative orthopaedic fracture patient, treatment should focus on anatomic reduction of the injury (if a fracture or dislocation) and its maintenance to prevent permanent effects and restore potential full functionality. Every attempt should be made to not only obtain reduction, but also maintain it throughout the period of fracture healing; even the smallest displacement, incongruity, or imperfect alignment may cause permanent issues with the affected limb.[2,3] Adequate pain management can be achieved through the use of pharmacologic therapies such as narcotics and other pain relievers. Other treatment modalities for orthopaedic fracture patients such as physical therapy, activity modification, ice, heat, and massage also contribute to the goals of adequate pain management and augmentation of functionality.

For orthopaedic patients with inflammatory conditions such as systemic lupus erythematosus or rheumatoid arthritis, treatment goals include reduction of pain, inflammation and stiffness, and preservation of the joints involved, specifically, the reduction or prevention of joint damage. This can be achieved pharmacologically with nonsteroidal anti-inflammatory drugs (NSAIDs), methotrexate, sulfasalazine, cyclosporine, and disease-modifying antirheumatic drugs. Strides should also be made in maintaining the functional ability of the joint and improving the joint's range of motion, which can be accomplished with the use of physical therapy.[4,5]

For conditions of overuse such as osteoarthritis or low back pain, the goals of treatment are reduction of pain and inflammation as well as the maintenance of functionality of involved joints. This, too, can be achieved pharmacologically with the use of NSAIDs and corticosteroid injections as well as through physical therapy.

Outcome expectations are determined by the nature of the orthopaedic injury itself and the process of healing. However, for a patient with an orthopaedic injury treated nonoperatively, outcome expectations should be based on being pain free and regaining pre-injury range of motion, with minimal or no limitations in ability to participate in exercise and sport. Patient outcome expectations are determined by the information patients are provided by physicians. Studies have demonstrated that relaying realistic goals and outcome expectations to patients not only contributes to the formation of patient expectations but can also optimally influence actual outcomes.[6-8]

II. PHYSICAL THERAPY

Physical therapy is the cornerstone of injury rehabilitation, and it has the ability to improve outcomes of orthopaedic injuries with or without surgical management, although this largely depends on the location and nature of the orthopaedic injury or condition.[9-14] This treatment modality aims for preinjury functional restoration through increasing muscle strength, joint mobility, patient endurance, and improving muscle coordination and control. Strength training programs involve movement against resistance. Increased endurance, which improves capacity for activities of daily living (ADLs), is achieved through endurance exercises that involve continuous activity like walking and swimming. Range of motion and flexibility can be improved by prolonged, low-intensity stretching exercises. Physical therapy employs various other modalities to treat orthopaedic injuries as well such as acupuncture/dry needling, iontophoresis, cryotherapy, electrotherapy, and hot and cold packs. Physiotherapy should be discontinued when goals have been met or there is lack of progress. Examples of physical therapy orders for a variety of nonoperative orthopaedic injuries and conditions are provided in Table 7-1.

III. SPLINTING AND CASTING (ALSO SEE CHAPTERS 8 AND 11)

Management of a wide variety of musculoskeletal conditions, such as fractures, sprains, strains, and even postoperative treatment of soft-tissue repairs, requires use of a splint (Figure 7-1) or cast (Figure 7-2)Both splints and casts share several common purposes: immobilization, reduction of pain, protection from further injury, and correction of a particular musculoskeletal injury. Casts are circumferential immobilizers that provide superior immobilization to splints. Casts are circumferential immobilizers that provide superior immobilization. They are generally reserved for definitive fracture management owing to their ability to facilitate healing by maintaining bones in appropriate alignment for extended periods of time. Additionally, casts are best used for an injury where edema has resolved or is considered insignificant to proper immobiliza-tion. A patient's extremity may not be ready for a cast owing to swelling until several days to weeks following acute injury. Splints, however, are noncircumferential devices used in acute scenarios that immobilize along three or fewer margins of an injured ex-tremity. This contributes to the ability of splints to accommodate

| TABLE 7-1 | Physical Therapy Orders for Common Nonoperative Orthopaedic Conditions |

Common Orthopaedic Conditions	Physical Therapy Orders
Ankle sprain	Acute: rest, ice, compression, and elevation of injured area Subacute: partial weight bearing, sagittal plane exercises and movement, isometric exercises of peroneal muscles Postacute: range of motion and muscle strengthening exercises, weight bearing, and proprioceptive training with progression to functional activities[20,22]
Ankle fracture	Acute: rest, ice, compression, and elevation of injured area Subacute: elevation, isometric exercises of immobilized muscles, strengthening of all other muscles Postacute: improvement of osteokinematic and arthrokinematic range of motion with progression to functional activities and weight bearing[9]
Trochanteric bursitis	Ultrasound, hydrocortisone-based coupling agent (phonophoresis), ionotophoresis, ice massage, and NSAIDs[23]
Low back pain	Core stability and dynamic stabilization exercises. Core stability exercises target the core of the body, including the lower back, trunk, and abdominal muscles (ie, sit-ups, back extensions, and abdominal muscles). Dynamic stabilization exercises keep the core steady as at least one extremity is moved (ie, exercise balls and balancing machines)[24]
Osteoarthritis of hip	Capsular stretch techniques and long axis distraction techniques for pain control and improvement in function[11,16]

TABLE 7-1	Physical Therapy Orders for Common Nonoperative Orthopaedic Conditions (*continued*)
Common Orthopaedic Conditions	**Physical Therapy Orders**
Impingement syndrome of the rotator cuff	Ice/heat, ultrasound/iontophoresis, massage, anterior–posterior gliding, long-term stretching, resistance exercises, and modification of activity[15]
Rheumatoid arthritis	Heat and cold, ultrasound, passive and active exercises for range of motion, dynamic exercise, rest with splinting, finger splinting, relaxation techniques[25]
Ankylosing spondylitis	Heat and cold, postural training, range of motion stretching, hydrotherapy[26]

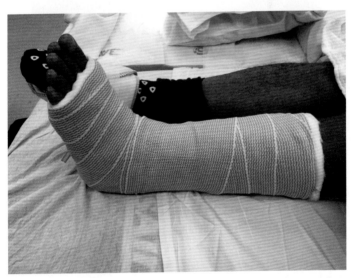

Figure 7-1 Short leg posterior splint. Image of patient in short leg posterior splint designed to keep the ankle in a neutral position.

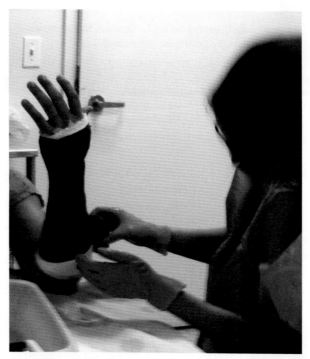

Figure 7-2 Short arm cast. Image of patient in short arm cast.

for swelling. This quality makes splints ideal for the management of a variety of acute musculoskeletal conditions in which edema inherent to the acute inflammatory response is imminent, such as acute fractures or sprains. Splints may also be used for the initial stabilization of reduced, displaced, or unstable fractures prior to orthopaedic surgical intervention.[15(pp494-502),16]

The use of casts and splints is generally limited to the short term, which maximizes the benefits while minimizing complications of their use. If continuously used or improperly placed, casts and splints cause excessive immobilization, which can lead to unintended outcomes such as chronic pain, joint stiffness, muscle atrophy, skin breakdown, or more severe complications. Subsequently, all patients who are placed in a splint or cast require careful monitoring to ensure proper healing and recovery.

Selection of a specific cast or splint varies based on the area of the body being treated and the stability of the injury. Indications and application techniques vary for each type of splint and cast commonly encountered.[15(pp404-405)]

IV. WEIGHT-BEARING STATUS AND ADVANCEMENT

Recommendations on weight bearing are variable and dependent upon the type of injury, the pathophysiology of the condition, and the age of the patient. For example, early weight bearing is encouraged in older patients with a stable orthopaedic injury. For a patient with an articular injury, the patient would be advanced to weight bearing after the healing process, which takes about 8 to 12 weeks and is assessed by serial radiograph. Immediate weight bearing, though dependent on the patient's comfort, is also an acceptable treatment for orthopaedic injuries that require conservative treatment as a result of minimal displacement. Immediate weight bearing can lead to union with minimal additional displacement.

Treatment of an orthopaedic injury in a nonoperative patient is dependent upon the condition being treated (Table 7-2). For a lower extremity fracture one would generally start making the patient nonweight bearing with slow but gradual advancement to partial and then full weight bearing. Overall, weight bearing status should be advanced as tolerated by the patient. It is best to confer with the treating physician with regard to weight-bearing status and advancement. Table 7-2 provides examples of weight-bearing recommendations for particular orthopaedic patients.

V. PAIN MANAGEMENT

Pain management is extremely important in the recovery process of all orthopaedic injuries. It also happens to be a major issue in the medical realm because of the reluctance of physicians to prescribe narcotic medication out of concern for addiction or disciplinary

TABLE 7-2	Weight-Bearing Recommendations for Nonoperative Orthopaedic Conditions
Nonoperative Orthopaedic Condition	**Weight-Bearing Recommendations**
Ankylosing spondylitis	Postural training and low-impact and low-intensity weight-bearing exercises such as swimming, yoga, and biking[27]
Rheumatoid arthritis	Low-intensity and low-impact weight bearing such as walking, swimming, and cycling[28,29]
Ankle sprain	Partial weight bearing in the subacute phase and full weight bearing in the postacute phase of healing[30]
Ankle fracture	Progression to full weight bearing in the postacute phase of healing[31]
Premenopausal osteoporosis	Bone loading exercises to increase bone mass such as walking, running, weight lifting, and hiking[32]
Osteoarthritis	Low-impact weight-bearing exercises like swimming and bicycling[33]

action by state medical boards. As a result, a common issue for patients with orthopaedic injuries requiring pain management is not achieving adequate pain control. Therefore, pain is assessed using a visual analog pain scale between 0 and 10—0 being no pain and 10 being the worst, most unbearable pain.[17] Pain is considered tolerable if the patient defines the pain as a 4 or less on the pain scale. It is important to note that tolerating pain is dependent upon the patient's personal pain threshold and tolerance and, therefore, is very subjective and individualized. Some patients may need more pain management than others because they have a lower threshold for pain. Constant communication with and feedback from the patient is required to develop an adequate personalized medication regimen that works.

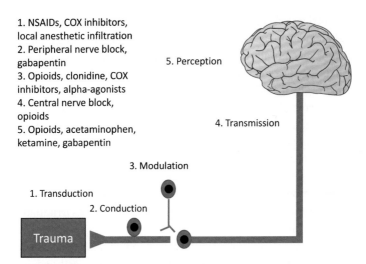

1. NSAIDs, COX inhibitors, local anesthetic infiltration
2. Peripheral nerve block, gabapentin
3. Opioids, clonidine, COX inhibitors, alpha-agonists
4. Central nerve block, opioids
5. Opioids, acetaminophen, ketamine, gabapentin

5. Perception

4. Transmission

3. Modulation

1. Transduction

2. Conduction

Trauma

Figure 7-3 **Multimodal analgesia.** Schematic demonstrating multimodal analgesia.

Pain management is predominantly achieved through pharmacologic therapy, and the best way to avoid an undermedicated patient is using a comprehensive, multimodal approach to pain management. Using several analgesics with mechanisms of action that address different points in the pain perception process will certainly better keep pain adequately controlled for the patient owing to the additive or synergistic analgesia. Figure 7-3 demonstrates multiple points in the pain perception process and lists the analgesics with mechanisms of action that target those points in the pain perception process.

For a nonoperative orthopaedic patient, oral narcotics, NSAIDs, and acetaminophen are used for pain control. NSAIDs in particular have been shown to reduce the need for narcotics owing to improved pain relief and a decrease in side effects of narcotics. Acetaminophen significantly relieves pain as well. Since its mechanism of action differs from that of narcotics, it can be used in conjunction with morphine and other narcotics. In this way, it can also reduce the requirement of narcotics, which can decrease the potential for abuse.

Corticosteroids are another anti-inflammatory medication for pain management and, depending on the condition being treated, can be given orally or by injection. For example, corticosteroids can be used to treat arthritis of a joint with injections but can be used orally for inflammatory orthopaedic conditions. Possible side effects of corticosteroids include acne, increased facial hair, moon-shaped facies, thin skin that easily bruises, the development of truncal body fat, increased appetite, weight gain, poor wound healing, headache, glaucoma, irregular menstrual periods, peptic ulcer, muscle weakness, osteoporosis, steroid-induced diabetes, and osteonecrosis. Patients that use corticosteroids may also experience various changes in mood and personality such as irritability, agitation, or depression.[18]

Gabapentin and pregabalin are calcium channel α2δ ligands used to manage neuropathic pain experienced by orthopaedic nonoperative patients. Typically, neuropathic pain is characterized as burning, tingling, or electric shocks triggered by light touch. It is a result of damage or dysfunction of the peripheral or central nociceptive pathways, leading to either a loss or an impairment in pain sensation. Side effects of gabapentin and pregabalin include sedation, dizziness, ataxia, and gastrointestinal side effects.[15(p157)]

There are other pain management options other than pharmacologic treatment such as physical therapy involving strengthening, stretching and traction, massage, and acupuncture. An alternate form of pain management is resting or stopping the activity that causes pain. For certain conditions, the cessation of pain-causing activity is a form of pain management that allows muscles, tendons, and joints time to rest and heal. Depending on the severity of the orthopaedic condition, rest may be prescribed.

VI. INITIATION OF IN-HOME CARE ARRANGEMENT

Determinants of the appropriate level of care include the functional limitations of the patient, the need for medical monitoring, social support, cognitive functioning, nursing needs, therapeutic disciplines required, and the ability to tolerate 3 hours of therapy a day. Home care and therapy have been demonstrated to be beneficial in that they improve functional outcomes, quality of life, and strength, and reduce the chance of accidental falls. Home care that focuses on daily living tasks, strength, endurance, and functional tasks, much like physical therapy, has been shown to be as effective as and is even more cost-effective than rehabilitation programs based in a center.

Persistent impairment and functional limitation may call for long-term home care and therapy. This includes decreased muscle strength, stability, flexibility, as well as overall decrease in ability to function. It has been statistically proven that patients who participate in home care and therapy experience significant improvements in muscle strength, stability, flexibility, and ability to function.

Home care and therapy are also an opportunity for patients to consider and improve upon their functional status, which may have been impaired by their orthopaedic injury or condition. ADLs are basic self-care tasks that are used to measure functional status. Functional status for patients can be assessed using the Katz Index of Independence in ADLs, which determines a patient's independence in the following tasks: bathing, dressing, toileting, transferring, continence, and feeding. A score of 0 or 1 is given for each task. If the patient requires no supervision, direction, or assistance with a task, he/she is given a 1 for that task. If, however, the patient requires supervision, direction, or assistance with a task, he/she is given a 0 for that task. The sum of the patient's scores for each of the 6 tasks represents the overall score, with an overall score of 6 indicating the patient is fully function. An overall score of 2 or less, on the other hand, indicates a patient with severe functional impairment A score of 6, one in each category, indicates that the patient is fully functional. A score of 4 demonstrates moderate impairment, and a score of 2 and below indicates severe functional impairment. Supervision needs are determined by the functional status of the patient, namely ambulation and self-care (ADLs). The more functionally impaired a patient is by his or her orthopaedic condition, the higher the patient's supervision needs.[19,20]

VII. RETURN TO SCHOOL, WORK, VOLUNTEERING, AND SPORT

For the orthopaedic patient treated non operatively, return to school is permitted as long as instructions are provided regarding the progression of activity allowed following orthopaedic injury and the patient's physical activity is carefully monitored to lessen the chance of reinjury and ensure full recovery. Therefore, patients returning to school should be excused from physical education class for some period of time as determined by the treating physician. Before returning to work and volunteering, patients should be provided with instructions for their supervisors detailing acceptable levels of activity that will allow for full recover. For the patient with orthopaedic conditions not requiring surgery, return to work can occur within several weeks depending on the type of work and what is expected of them. It should be kept in mind that work requiring manual labor is usually delayed in someone with an orthopaedic injury. Return to sport with low-impact exercises is preferred, such as elliptical biking or golf followed by progressive return to full activities over time.

VIII. DRIVING EXPECTATIONS

Patients frequently ask when they will have the ability to resume driving a motor vehicle following their orthopaedic injuries and rely on a physician's permission for return to normal daily activities. Being able to drive for many provides a level of independence and functionality for patients, which is why driving is considered as an activity of daily living. The ability to operate a motor vehicle safely is a multifactorial process that involves the integration of physical, neurologic, and cognitive abilities including the abilities to brake, steer, throttle, and see. Orthopaedic injuries often interfere with a patient's ability to drive, particularly as a result of pain, limited range of motion, limited force, and altered movement patterns of the extremities needed.[2]

Ultimately, driving recommendations are given as they can be tolerated by the patient, with the recommendations being dependent upon the location of the injury and whether the injury is transient or permanent. Accommodations can be made to assist patients' return to driving an automobile. There is no medical clearance from the orthopaedic perspective to provide a patient. A discussion of expectations and needs should be had with the patient and physician to assess specific limitations that may affect the ability to safely operate a motor vehicle.[21]

REFERENCES

1. Hughes JL, Weber H, Willenegger H, Kuner EH. Evaluation of ankle fractures: non-operative and operative treatment. *Clin Orthop Relat Res.* 1979;138:111-119.

2. Iserson KV. Orthopedics. In: Iserson KV, eds. *Improvised Medicine: Providing Care in Extreme Environments.* 2nd ed. New York, NY: McGraw-Hill; 2016. http://accessmedicine.mhmedical.com/content.aspx?bookid=1728&Sectionid=115698090. Accessed October 19, 2016.

3. Thomas BJ, Fu FH, Muller B, et al. Orthopedic surgery. In: Brunicardi F, Andersen DK, Billiar TR, et al, eds. *Schwartz's Principles of Surgery.* 10th ed. New York, NY: McGraw-Hill; 2014. http://accessmedicine.mhmedical.com/content.aspx?bookid=980&Sectionid=59610885. Accessed October 19, 2016.

4. Moreland LW, Canella A. General principles of management of rheumatoid arthritis in adults. In: Post TW, ed. *UpToDate.* Waltham, MA: UpToDate; 2016.

5. Wallace DJ. Overview of the management and prognosis of systemic lupus erythematosus in adults. In: Post TW, ed. *UpToDate.* Waltham, MA: UpToDate; 2016.

6. Henn RF III, Kang L, Tashjian RZ, Green A. Patients' preoperative expectations predict the outcome of rotator cuff repair. *J Bone Joint Surg Am.* 2007;89(9):1913-1919.

7. Waljee J, Mcglinn EP, Sears ED, Chung KC. Patient expectations and patient-reported outcomes in surgery: a systematic review. *Surgery.* 2014;155(5):799-808.

8. Schouten R, Lewkonia P, Noonan VK, et al. Expectations of recovery and functional outcomes following thoracolumbar trauma: an evidence-based medicine process to determine what surgeons should be telling their patients. *J Neurosurg Spine.* 2015;22(1):101-111.

9. Evgeniadis G, Beneka A, Malliou P, Godolias G. Effects of pre- or postoperative therapeutic exercise on the quality of life, before and after total knee arthroplasty for osteoarthritis. *J Back Musculoskelet Rehabil.* 2008;21(3):161-169.

10. De Carlo MS, Sell KE. The effects of the number and frequency of physical therapy treatments on selected outcomes of treatment in patients with anterior cruciate ligament reconstruction. *J Orthop Sports Phys Ther.* 1997;26(6):332-339.

11. Di Fabio RP, Boissonnault W. Physical therapy and health-related outcomes for patients with common orthopaedic diagnoses. *J Orthop Sports Phys.* 1998;27(3):219-230.

12. Kay TM, Gross A, Goldsmith CH, et al. Exercises for mechanical neck disorders. *Cochrane Database of Systematic Rev.* 2005;(3):CD0042520.

13. Persson LC, Carlsson CA, Carlsson JY. Long-lasting cervical radicular pain managed with surgery, physiotherapy, or a cervical collar. *Spine.* 1997;22(7):751-758.

14. Childress MA, Becker BA. Nonoperative management of cervical radiculopathy. *Am Fam Physician.* 2016;93(9):746-754.

15. Donatelli R, Wooden MJ. *Orthopaedic Physical Therapy.* New York, NY: Churchill Livingstone; 2001.

16. Maughan KL. Ankle sprain. In: Post TW, ed. *UpToDate.* Waltham, MA: UpToDate; 2017.

17. Rand SE, Goerlich C, Marchand K, Jablecki N. The physical therapy prescription. *Am Fam Physician.* 2007;76(11):1661-1666.

18. Reiman MP, Matheson JW. Restricted hip mobility: clinical suggestions for self-mobilization and muscle re-education. *Int J Sports Phys Ther.* 2013;8(5):729-740.

19. Schur PH, Ravinder NM, Gibofsky A. Nonpharmacologic therapies and preventive measures for patients with rheumatoid arthritis. In: Post TW, ed. *UpToDate.* Waltham, MA: UpToDate; 2016.

20. Yu DT. Assessment and treatment of ankylosing spondylitis in adults. In: Post TW, ed. *UpToDate.* Waltham, MA: UpToDate; 2016.

21. Doherty GM. *Current Diagnosis & Treatment Surgery.* 14th ed. New York, NY: McGraw-Hill; 2015. http://accessmedicine.mhmedical.com.ezproxy.med.nyu.edu/content.aspx?bookid=1202§ionid=71527086. Accessed October 18, 2016.

22. Boyd AS, Benjamin HJ, Asplund C. Splints and casts: indications and methods. *Am Fam Physician.* 2009;80(5):491-499.

23. Schur PH, Maini RN, Gibofsky A. Nonpharmacologic therapies and preventive measures for patients with rheumatoid arthritis. In: Post TW, ed. *UpToDate.* Waltham, MA: UpToDate, 2016.

24. Westby MD, Wade JP, Rangno KK, et al. A randomized controlled trial to evaluate the effectiveness of an exercise program in women with rheumatoid arthritis taking low dose prednisone. *J Rheumatol.* 2000;27(7):1674-1680.

25. Becker CB, Cohen A. Evaluation and treatment of premenopausal osteoporosis. In: Post TW, ed. *UpToDate.* Waltham, MA: UpToDate; 2016.

26. Kalunian KC. Nonpharmacologic therapy of osteoarthritis. In: Post TW, ed. *UpToDate.* Waltham, MA: UpToDate; 2016.

27. McCaffery M, Beebe A. *Pain: Clinical Manual for Nursing Practice.* Baltimore, MD: V.V. Mosby Company; 1993.

28. Rabow MW, Pantilat SZ. Palliative care & pain management. In: Papadakis MA, McPhee SJ, Rabow MW, eds. *Current Medical Diagnosis & Treatment 2017.* New York, NY: McGraw-Hill; 2016. http://accessmedicine.mhmedical.com/content.aspx?bookid=1843&Sectionid=135698406. Accessed October 18, 2016.

29. Rathmell JP, Fields HL. *Pain: Pathophysiology and Management.* In: Kasper D, Fauci A, Hauser S, Longo D, Jameson J, Loscalzo J, eds. *Harrison's Principles of Internal Medicine.* 19 ed. New York, NY: McGraw-Hill; 2015. http://accessmedicine.mhmedical.com/content.aspx?bookid=1130&Sectionid=79724180. Accessed October 18, 2016.

30. Reuben DB, Leonard SD. Office-based assessment of the older adult. In: Post TW, ed. *UpToDate.* Waltham, MA: UpToDate; 2016.

31. Miller CA. Katz Index of independence in activities of daily living. *Geriatr Nurs.* 2000;21(2):109.

32. Egol KA, Sheikhazadeh A, Koval KJ. Braking function after complex lower extremity trauma. *J Trauma.* 2008;65(6):1435-1438.

33. Sheikhzadeh A, Pinto V. Medical aspects of fitness to drive: the human factors role. *Ergon Des: Q Hum Factors Applic.* 2014;22(1):16-22.

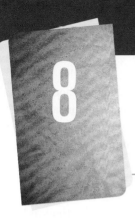

8

NAVIGATING THE OPERATING ROOM

David Kugelman and Kenneth A. Egol

I. GREETING THE PATIENT

As an orthopaedic provider, the operating room may be very familiar to you, but it is a unique and often intimidating place for patients. This may be their first elective operation or an emergency surgery following a traumatic incident. No matter the reason, the patient is our number one priority and should be greeted politely and made as comfortable as possible prior, during, and following an operation.

Hygiene and Proper Introduction

When initially greeting a patient, the most important thing to do is to first wash your hands followed by a polite introduction.[1] Dress professionally and avoid wearing religious jewelry or political buttons that may interfere with a patient's beliefs. The patient is often meeting an entire team in the hours before an operation. It is appropriate to greet the patient with your name, professional or student title, and role on his/her health care team.

Interview the Patient

After the formal meet and greet, the next step should be conducting a proper patient interview and obtaining a thorough medical history.[2] Important information to review includes: the patient's past medical conditions, surgical history, and prior anesthesia complications if applicable. Verify blood type, current medications, and allergies.

After this review, assess the patient's general state of health including mental capacity, emotional state, time of last meal, and last insulin dose if diabetic. Perform a review of systems, including a thorough menstrual and obstetric history for female patients. Inquire about recent events that may have occurred in a hospital stay or at home.

In addition, identify risk factors for communicable diseases such as hepatitis and HIV.

Discussion of the Procedure

During this interview, it is important to make the patient as comfortable as possible. This may be a difficult moment for the patient. In explaining your role on the team, you can let the patient know the plan for the rest of the operative day. Inform them of the plan of care such as anesthesia to be administered, the operative procedure, and estimated time of the procedure. At the end of the conversation, ask the patient if they have any further questions you or another member of the medical team may be able to answer. Make sure the patient has not eaten or had anything to drink for at least 8 hours prior to the procedure.

Physical Examination

A review of pertinent history and an updated physical examination should be conducted to assess changes since the preoperative physical examination.[3] Begin with obtaining vital signs. Perform proper cardiovascular, pulmonary, and abdominal examinations to assess for murmurs, heart rate, abnormal breath sounds, and tenderness. Assess for changes to skin integrity such as wounds or rashes and rule out a visible infection. Any changes should be documented in the medical record (refer to Chapter 4).

Chart Review, Imaging, and Labs

It may be important to fill in any gaps in the history and physical with a proper chart review including labs and imaging. Review past medical and/or surgical notes in order to see the full scope of the surgical patient. Pertinent labs and information include the following[3]: CBC, BMP, input/output, microbiology cultures, pathology reports, appropriate imaging, allergies, allied health updates (PT, OT), and medications.

While escorting the patient into the operating room, make the patient feel as comfortable as possible. As the patient enters the operating room, everyone should introduce himself or herself to the patient and then help team members properly position the patient.

II. ROOM PREPARATION

When helping prepare the operating room, it is once again of extreme importance to ensure proper hygiene measures are taken. Thoroughly wash your hands and ensure clean scrubs are worn. Be sure to wear shoe covers, have all hair enclosed in a surgical cap, and wear a mask to prevent contaminating the operating field. The mask should fit snugly around the nose and mouth to filter the air through the mask, rather than from the sides. The Association of Operating Room Nurses and The Center for Medicare & Medicaid Services recommend head coverings, such as bouffant hats, in the operating room.[4] Covering of the head and skin is of upmost importance, as humans may shed up to one million microorganisms every day.[5] These microorganisms as well as other breaks in sterility can lead to the complication of postoperative infections; therefore, the hygiene measures described above should be taken extremely seriously.

Staff involved in hip and knee replacements take even further hygienic precautions, through the use of surgical helmet systems, also known as "space suits" or "hoods" (Figure 8-1). The surgical helmet system comprises a helmet with personal airflow, which is covered with a sterile visor mask hood. These space suits have been shown to reduce infections following arthroplasty. This special headwear is designed to limit airborne bacterial contaminates.[6]

Familiarize Yourself with the Operating Room

Introduce yourself to the operating room staff and be sure to explain your role in the surgical team. The scrub tech and circulator will be arranging the equipment in the operating room in a sterile manner. Be aware of your surroundings and keep appropriate distance from

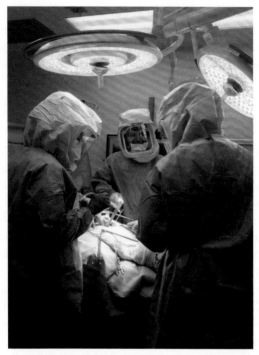

Figure 8-1 **Surgical helmet systems ("space suits" or "hoods") worn by the operating staff in joint arthroplast.** Image demonstrating surgical helmet systems ("space suits" or "suits") worn by operating staff in joint arthroplasty cases.

the sterile fields. Do not be timid in notifying the operating room staff if you suspect that the field or an instrument may have been contaminated. In addition, it is courteous to provide the scrub tech with your gown and sterile gloves.

Make Sure Imaging Is Available in the Room

For each procedure, it is important to review the patient's imaging in the operating room. Therefore, it is imperative that films can be displayed on screens in the OR or that hard copy films are available for review. Preoperative planning for joint replacements may be accompanied by the use of a digital template. These templates

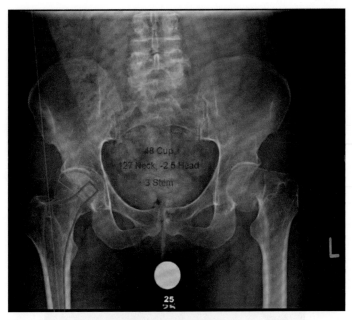

Figure 8-2 Templating for total hip arthroplasty. Image demonstrating sample template for total hip arthroplasty procedure.

are designed for specific implants and are placed over the patient's preoperative imaging, in order to plan for the size and type of surgical implant needed (Figure 8-2).

OR Table Preparation

There are a variety of accessories that are used to prepare the OR table. Arm boards, lithotomy stirrups, lateral positioning bars, and posts attach to the table. Gel pads, positioners, pillows, bean bags, foam, and other padding devices are needed to prevent pressure ulcers (Figure 8-3). Pillows are also commonly used to prevent pressure ulcer formation (Figure 8-4). These devices keep a normal capillary interface with pressures at 32 mm Hg or less. Pay special attention to bony prominences as they are at greater risk for developing ulcers. As many as 25% of postoperative pressure ulcers may be induced from the OR.[7]

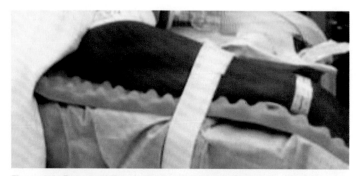

Figure 8-3 **Foam padding device used to prevent pressure ulcers.** Image demonstrating foam padding device used to prevent pressure ulcers.

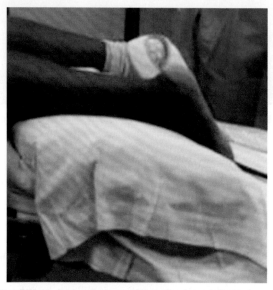

Figure 8-4 **Pillows in use, for prevention of pressure ulcers.** Image demonstrating use of pillows to prevent pressure ulcers.

Time-out

A time-out is a universal patient safety protocol performed by the surgical team to prevent errors in surgery.[8] Before the patient is ready to undergo anesthesia, a time-out is run by a designated member of the surgical team (Figure 8-5). The purpose of the time-out is to

UNIVERSAL PROTOCOL GUIDE/RN Prompted Time Out	
PRE-INCISION/ PROCEDURE TIME OUT:	
SURGEON CALLS TIME OUT, ALL PAUSE, Team Members Introduce Themselves	
Prompt	**Response**
Pt Name and DOB	Surgeon or RN + Anesthesia confirms in EHR
Procedure	Surgeon states + RN compares w/consent
Side/ Site Marking	Surgeon states + All Team Members confirm and visualize marking (including special purpose band)
Position Safe & Correct?	Surgeon
Allergies	Anesthesia Care Provider
Antibiotics	Anesthesia Care Provider + RN confirms documentation in EHR
DVT prophylaxis initiated?	Surgeon (yes or NA) (if SCD's, RN ensures SCD machine is on and tubing connected)
Neutral Zone Established	Scrub identifies location of Neutral Zone for hands free passing (if applicable)
Implants	Surgeon
If Implant, Expiration Date	RN confirms expiration date(s) valid
Imaging needed in room?	Surgeon (RN confirms name & DOB on image displayed in room)
Anticipated Specimens?	Surgeon
If "Yes", any special handling of specimens?	Surgeon
If a Central Line was placed in the OR/Procedure Room prior to Time Out Dual verification that the GuideWire was removed	Anesthesia & RN

Figure 8-5 **Example of an OR checklist used to complete the "time-out" protocol.**

RN state: ENTERING FIRE SAFETY TIME OUT	
Procedure above or below xiphoid?	Surgeon
Closed or open system?	Anesthesia Care Provider
If open delivery, is 02 > 29% in a procedure ABOVE xiphoid? If so, discuss use of LMA, ET. If proceed w/open 02, must be isolated by incise drape.	
Prep Solution Used?	Surgeon, if alcohol based prep, state dry time > 3 min
Ignition sources?	Surgeon/ Team (name all ie laser, ESU, light cord, etc)
Fire Extinguisher location	RN
Fire Risk (from EHR)	RN (Low: 1, 2 High: 3)
If HIGH, must discuss fire safety plan	**Each Team Member state plan and role**
Did Briefing Occur with the Team?	Surgeon MUST CONFIRM discussion took place w/ Attending Anesthesiologist, nursing, and Team Members
Would anyone like to add to the briefing?	All Team Members
RN state: IF ANYONE HAS ANY CONCERNS AT ANY TIME, SPEAK UP	
Everyone Agree?	All Team Members

Figure 8-5 (*continued*)

make sure the entire team is in agreement regarding the correct patient, side and location of surgery, all equipment is available, medications are given, and fire safety has been reviewed. A time-out involves immediate members of the surgical team such as the surgeons, physician assistants (PAs), nurse practitioners, anesthesia providers, circulating nurses, operating room technicians, students, and other members present in the operating room. The time-out should involve verification of the patient's name and date of birth, procedure, and surgical site. Time-out needs to be performed for each individual procedure if the patient is undergoing more than one.

III. POSITIONING AND PATIENT PREPARATION

The patient's position should provide the surgeon with the best possible exposure. The position should not compromise the patient's circulatory, respiratory, musculoskeletal, or neurologic function. While under anesthesia, the patient cannot relate any discomfort in positioning; therefore, it is important to follow normal anatomy and positioning as not to overstretch muscles, tendons, or joints. Venous and arterial lines should be easily accessible because anesthesia may also cause peripheral dilation, decreased cardiac output, and hypotension.

General Positioning Principles

Before transferring the patient, make sure the stretcher is in a locked position.[9,10] Anatomic alignment of the patient on the OR table should be maintained as closely as possible. This can be facilitated through placement of pillows between the legs if in a lateral position or posterior to the knees if supine.

It is of critical importance that all bony prominences be properly padded to prevent pressure ulcers. Keep anatomic alignment by assuring joints not be moved past normal range of motion. Lastly, secure the patient with straps or tape when on the OR table.

General Patient Positions

Patient positioning depends on the limb being operated on, the procedure being performed, and the approach that is taken (Figures 8-6 to 8-10).[9] Ask the attending beforehand how they would like the patient positioned. The following are four common positions used in orthopaedic surgery:

1. Supine: place patient flat on back with arms outstretched at less than 90 degrees or placed on side (Figure 8-6).
2. Prone: place patient face down; if endotracheal intubation is needed, this is first done in a supine position and the patient is then turned over (Figure 8-7).

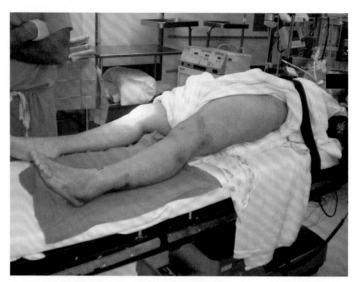

Figure 8-6 **Demonstration of supine positioning.** Image demonstrating patient in the supine position.

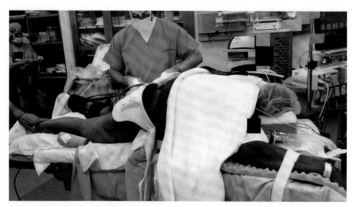

Figure 8-7 **Demonstration of prone positioning.** Image demonstrating patient in the prone position.

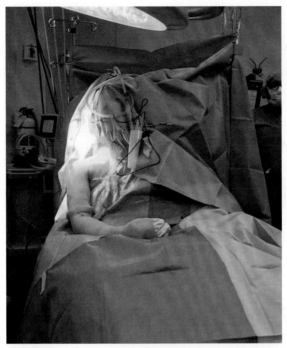

Figure 8-8 **Demonstration of the sitting (beach chair) positioning.** Image demonstrating patient in the sitting (beach chair) position.

3. Sitting (beach chair): table is elevated to 60 degrees, and the extremity is off the edge of the table allowing access to both the anterior and posterior shoulders (Figure 8-8).
4. Jackknife: place patient in prone position with torso and legs slightly lowered (Figure 8-9).
5. Lateral: Place patient in lateral decubitus position on a beanbag or in a lateral positioner (Figure 8-10).

Tourniquet

In surgery on the limbs, a tourniquet is often applied to create a bloodless field. Test the tourniquet before placing it on the patient, and make sure it is padded to prevent blistering of skin. Tourniquets

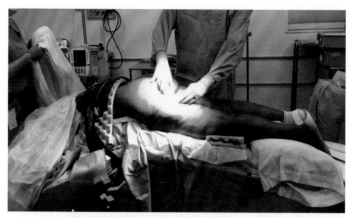

Figure 8-9 Demonstration of jackknife positioning. Image demonstrating patient in the jackknife position.

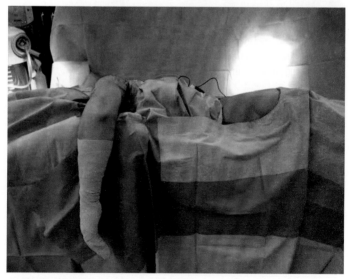

Figure 8-10 Demonstration of lateral positioning. Image demonstrating patient in the lateral position.

are usually applied to the limb prior to sterile prep, but may also be applied to the prepped limb sterilely during the procedure. Following the time-out, drain the limb of blood by elevating the limb for 3 to 5 minutes or applying a compression bandage. Pressure of the inflated tourniquet varies but should be greater than twice the systolic BP for most patients.[9] In children and hypertensive patients, the tourniquet should be inflated 50% above the systolic pressure.[9] Tourniquets should be applied for a maximum time of 2 to 2½ hours.[9] Caution should be used when applying tourniquets in patients who have compromised circulation such as sickle cell disease.

Prepping and Draping

All patients undergoing surgical intervention must undergo aseptic preparation of the skin. There are different types of antibacterial solutions that are commonly used for aseptic preparation of the skin. Chlorhexidine gluconate is a common aqueous-based solution, which works by disrupting bacterial cell membranes. Aqueous-based iodophors, such as Betadine, release free iodine, which acts as an antiseptic through destroying microbial proteins and DNA. Alcohol-based solutions, such as DuraPrep, contain iodine povacrylex and isopropyl alcohol. They are commonly used in orthopaedic procedures, because it is applied in one step, has a dry time of a minimum of 3 minutes, and leaves a water-insoluble film on the skin surface that keeps its antimicrobial activity for as long as 48 hours. DuraPrep enhances surgical drape to skin adhesion, which may limit the spread of organisms from the patient to the surgical field.[11] Following the aseptic preparation of the skin, the operative site is draped out and all areas outside are not considered sterile.

IV. INTRAOPERATIVE IMAGING

As discussed previously, appropriate imaging of the patient's pathology and anatomy should be put on display when preparing the operating room. Imaging should be kept on display during the procedure as well.

Many orthopaedic procedures use intraoperative fluoroscopy. This is a major aspect of trauma cases when reduction and fixation must be constantly assessed. Some procedures use postoperative fluoroscopy or plain X-ray as well when the patient is still sedated. This includes trauma procedures involving hardware placement and joint arthroplasty. When intraoperative imaging is expected, all staff in the room are required to wear lead shielding. If an individual will be scrubbing into a case, they must put on a lead shield and thyroid shield prior to handwashing and being gowned. Physicians and staff that are often in operating rooms where fluoroscopy is used are recommended to use radiation monitors to track their exposure to intraoperative radiation. This is common in fields such as orthopaedic trauma, in which intraoperative fluoroscopy is frequently used in order to visualize the reduction and fixation of a fracture.

Patient positioning is essential to obtaining easy and accessible radiographs, thereby decreasing operating time and allowing for accurate assessment of reduction and implant placement.

Upper Extremity

Shoulder

Proximal humerus and clavicle fractures are treated with the patient in a beach chair position.[10] Images can be obtained by placing a bump placed under the medial scapular border of the injured side, which slightly turns the patient to the contralateral side. The head should remain in neutral rotation with slight flexion to secure the airway. The image intensifier is often positioned above the patient to obtain proper anteroposterior (AP) and axillary views of the proximal humerus (Figure 8-11).

Clavicle images should be obtained with the airway tube facing the contralateral side so as to not obstruct the injured side. The image intensifier is also brought from the contralateral side (Figure 8-12).

Humerus and Elbow

The patient may be in the lateral or supine position depending on the exposure needed for the case. Positioning of the patient is

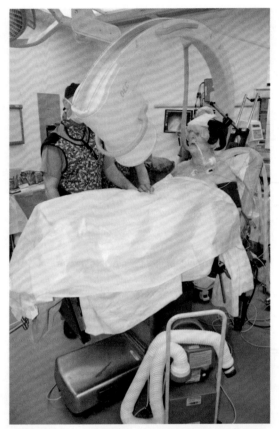

Figure 8-11 **Intraoperative imaging of proximal humerus fracture.**

chosen in response to fracture pattern and surgeon preference. The posterior approach of the arm is taken for procedures involving the humeral shaft, distal humerus, and olecranon. The patient is in the lateral decubitus position and is stabilized with a bean bag. For this approach, the affected extremity may be hung over an armrest for added support and to help facilitate the reduction. It is also important to note that an axillary roll should be placed in the axilla of the noninjured arm, in order to reduce the risk of a brachial plexus traction injury (Figure 8-13).

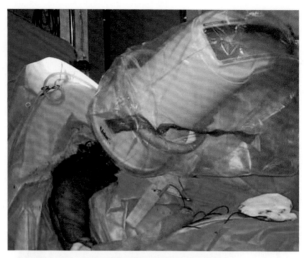

Figure 8-12 **Intraoperative imaging of clavicle fracture.**

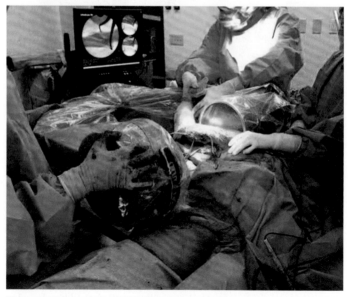

Figure 8-13 **Intraoperative image of arm and elbow using posterior approach.**

A direct lateral or anterolateral approach is often used for humeral shaft, distal humerus, radial head, proximal radius, and proximal ulna fractures. The patient is supine during this approach and the affected extremity is often placed upon a hand table (Figure 8-14).

In both positions, the image intensifier is brought in from the injured side to obtain AP and lateral views.

Wrist and Hand

Patients with wrist and hand fractures are placed in supine position with the injured extremity on a hand table or arm board. This is the most common positioning for hand procedures and fractures of the

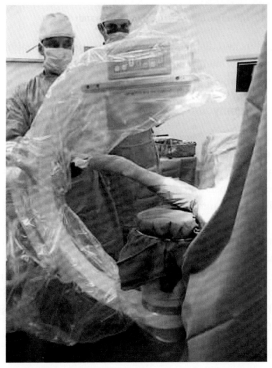

Figure 8-14 **Intraoperative imaging of arm and elbow using direct lateral and/or anterolateral approaches.**

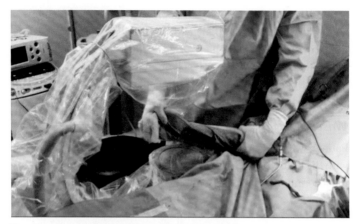

Figure 8-15 **Intraoperative imaging of wrist/hand.**

distal radius and distal ulna. The forearm may be manipulated in order to provide lateral and AP views. The image intensifier is brought in from the same side to obtain AP and lateral views (Figure 8-15).

Lower Extremity

Pelvis

An anterior approach to the pelvis has the patient supine on the operating table with a bump under the small of the patient's back to increase lordosis and obtain proper sacral imaging.[10] The image intensifier is brought from the contralateral side of the injured pelvis. For inlet views, the machine is tilted in a caudal fashion, and images are accurate when the upper sacral vertebrae appear circular in shape. The image intensifier is put in a cephalad position to obtain the outlet view, and images are accurate when the superior pubic symphysis is superimposed on the vertebral S2 body. Lateral views are obtained and verified when landmarks such as iliocortical density are in view (Figure 8-16).

Acetabulum

A posterior approach has the patient prone with the hip extended and knee flexed between 80 and 90 degrees. The image intensifier

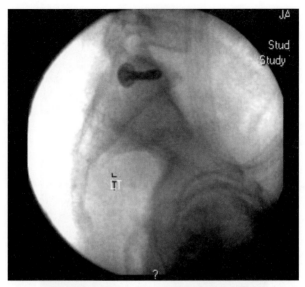

Figure 8-16 Intraoperative image of lateral sacral view demonstrating screw in the S1 body below the iliocortical density.

is brought from the contralateral side to obtain AP and Judet views (45 degree oblique images). An anterior approach has the patient supine with the hip slightly flexed in order to relax the iliopsoas muscles and the femoral nerve. The image intensifier is brought in from the contralateral side. A percutaneous approach has the patient in a supine position. The image intensifier is brought in from the contralateral side (Figure 8-17).

Hip and Femoral Shaft

For hip fractures, the patient is placed in a supine position on a fracture table with the injured limb secured in a boot (Figure 8-18). Secure the patient with a padded perineal post then scissor and secure the contralateral leg or place the contralateral leg on a padded leg positioner. Rotate the torso to the contralateral side and secure the ipsilateral arm across the patient's chest to the contralateral side of the table. Bring the image intensifier from the

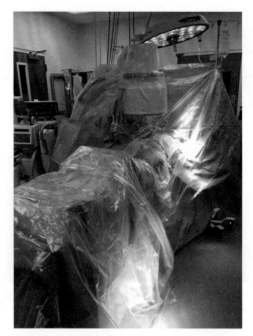

Figure 8-17 **Intraoperative imaging of acetabulum fracture.**

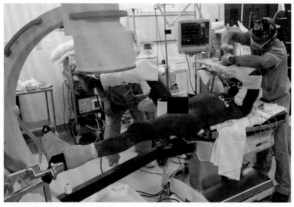

Figure 8-18 **Fracture table.** Image depicting patient positioned on a fracture table.

contralateral side and position it under the table for cross-table lateral views of the hip.

For femoral shaft fractures, place the patient in a supine position on a radiolucent or fracture table. If a fracture table is used, secure the contralateral leg to a metal post of the table. Bring the image intensifier from the contralateral side. Use a sterile bump to elevate the injured extremity out of the plane of the uninjured extremity for the lateral view.

For hip arthroplasty, several approaches may be used, including: anterior, anterolateral and posterior. Positioning for these procedures may depend on prosthesis choice and surgeon preference. For the anterolateral approach, the patient is placed in a supine position where the buttock of the surgical side hangs over the operating table. The table is then tilted toward the contralateral side. For the posterior approach, the patient is placed in a lateral position with the affected limb facing up. Place a cushion under the lateral malleolus and knee of the bottom leg along with a pillow between the knees. For the anterior approach, the patient is placed in a supine position. For the lateral approach, the patient is placed in a supine position. For postoperative imaging, bring the image intensifier in from the contralateral side so AP and lateral views can be obtained.

Knee Procedures

For fractures of the distal femur, tibial plateau, and patella, the patient is placed in a supine position. Place a bump under the injured extremity for internal rotation. Bring the image intensifier in from the contralateral side to obtain AP and lateral views. Use a sterile bump to elevate the injured extremity out of the plane of the uninjured extremity for the lateral view (Figure 8-19).

Knee arthroplasty can be performed using numerous approaches which all require the same patient positioning. The patient is placed in a supine position with cushioning under the thigh on the side of the affected knee. Avoid placing cushioning under the popliteal

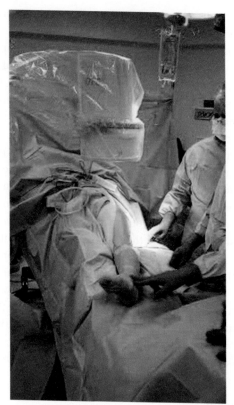

Figure 8-19 **Intraoperative imaging of knee.**

fossa as it may compress the popliteal artery and posterior joint capsule against the femur or tibia. Remove the end of the operating table to allow knee flexion during the procedure. For postoperative imaging, bring the image intensifier in from the contralateral side so AP and lateral views can be obtained.

Tibial Shaft

The patient is placed in the supine position. Use a radiolucent triangle to hyperflex the knee if a standard approach is used or semiextend the knee if a suprapatellar approach is used. Bring the image intensifier underneath the table to obtain lateral views for visual confirmation of safe reamer and nail passage.

Foot and Ankle Procedures

If internal rotation of the affected extremity is needed, the patient is placed in the supine position with a bump under the ipsilateral hip. Bring the image intensifier in from the contralateral side to obtain AP, lateral, and oblique views of the ankle or foot. If extension of the affected extremity is needed, the patient is placed in the prone position with a bump under the ipsilateral hip. Bring the image intensifier in from the contralateral side to obtain AP, lateral, and oblique views of the ankle or foot.

V. INTRAOPERATIVE ASSIST

As a practitioner, you will be assisting the lead surgeon and help him/her execute the procedure as efficiently and safely as possible.[12] This involves anticipating the surgeon's movement through knowledge of the procedure. In addition to a focus on what is currently taking place during a surgery, you should focus on the next step of the procedure as well—what instrument and maneuver are needed to accomplish the current and next step. Four different skills that you may be asked to perform in the OR will be discussed: retraction, suturing and knot-tying, providing traction, and dissection.

Retracting

Retractors are used to gain good visual exposure when surgery is being performed. Exposure is one of the most important aspects of surgical assist. Inadequate exposure is one of the most common causes of surgical failure. Therefore, it is important to know which operative approach will be used as you prepare for the case. In addition to retraction for exposure, it is important to keep the field clean of blood using gauze and suction. Make sure fingers are out of a surgeon's line of sight. Be aware of the tissues you are retracting.

Exposed tissues can contribute to desiccation and fluid loss; be sure to keep tissues moist with saline-soaked gauze and/or irrigation. Handle tissues gently with forceps and hands. It is important to release the retraction during breaks or when procedures are not actively being performed.

Examples of handheld retractors:

1. Army-Navy and Senn retractors are used for retraction of superficial tissue.
2. Richardson retractor is used for retraction of tissues within cavities and for deep incisions.
3. Deaver and Harrington retractors are used for viscera and abdominal wall retraction and delicate organs, respectively.

Suturing and Knot-Tying

Suturing and knot-tying are an extremely important aspect of surgery that may be performed on occasion by a first-assist. This takes a great deal of practice that should be done outside the operating room on suture boards or pigs' feet. Knot-tying can be easily practiced on a knot tie board or even one's belt loop. When practicing, pay attention to the following:

Create a secure knot without strangulation of tissue. Use pads of fingers when tightening knots to prevent cuts. When cutting sutures, slide the tips of the scissors down the strands to the point where they will be cut, and cut at a 45-degree angle. For external nonabsorbing suture, leave 4 to 5 mm of suture tail for an easy removal. Common suture techniques include simple interrupted, subcutaneous, horizontal mattress, and vertical mattress suturing (Figure 8-20).

Traction

Providing intraoperative, manual traction allows continuous exposure of underlying structures when dissecting tissue layers and contributes to less force being used for cleavage. Gently pull the tissues in opposite directions. The surgeon will pull on one side and make the cut while the assistant provides traction in the opposite direction.

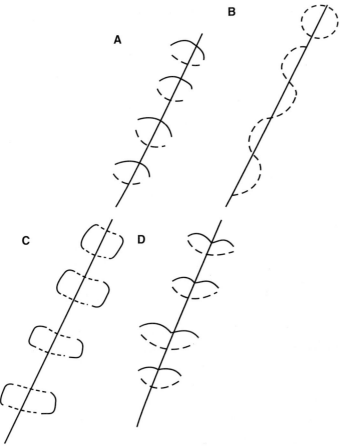

Figure 8-20 Common suturing techniques. A: simple interrupted sutures. B: subcutaneous sutures. C: Horizontal mattress sutures. D: Vertical mattress sutures. Key: Solid lines are visible and on the exterior of the skin, while the dotted lines are in, or under, the incision.

Dissection

Follow anatomic planes when possible. Never dissect or cut any tissue that cannot be visualized. Blunt dissection with a nonsharp instrument is used for separation of loose tissue around neuro-vascular structures.

VI. CASTING AND SPLINTING (DETAILS IN CHAPTERS 7 AND 11)

Splints are often applied in the operating room following an open reduction and internal fixation. The purpose of casts and splints is to immobilize, protect, and, if necessary, reduce a fracture or dislocation. Splints are used to immobilize an immediate injury that may be accompanied by edema. They immobilize along three or fewer margins, whereas casts immobilize throughout the entire circumference of an extremity. Splints may be taken off once the acute inflammatory phase is complete and swelling is resolved or negligible—at this point, a cast may be used for proper immobilization.

Casting and Splinting Considerations

Padding, elastic bandages, and stockinettes should be appropriate in length and fit;[12] do not make too tight because circulation may be compromised. Plaster should not overlap circumferentially.

In regard to padding, the following steps should be taken: Roll the padding in the distal to proximal direction. Overlap each new layer of padding or cast tape with half the prior, with a minimum of two layers. Make sure to apply extra padding to bony prominences. The padding should be taut, but do not apply too much where the padding tears. For splint application, wet the material with room temperature water and wring out any excess water (dry towel may be used to damp dry). If the water is too warm, there is a quicker set time of the material; in addition, the material releases heat and this can cause skin burns. If using plaster, the material may shrink when wet. Keep in mind beforehand for appropriate fitting that the plaster layer should be 12 to 15 layers thick for the usual adult—6-inch width for thigh, 4- to 6-inch width for legs and arms, or 2- to 4-inch width for forearm and wrist.

For cast application, wet the cast tape or plaster with room temperature water and leave material wet or slightly wet. Somewhat damp material is beneficial because, if too dry, the set time will be quickened, just as occurs with warmer water. Apply appropriate tension by unrolling cast material. Fiberglass may be used instead of plaster; it is more resistant to moisture and breakdown, but is more difficult to mold. It also has decreased chance of thermal injury.

Casting and Splinting Complications

The following are some of the complications that may arise following extremity casting and splinting: Loss of reduction, pressure necrosis (as quickly as in 2 hours following application), and compartment syndrome. Univalving and bivalving a circumferential cast can reduce pressures by 30% and 60%, respectively; cutting of casts and splitting of underlying Webril padding reduce pressure further. Using "cast spreaders" minimizes contact pressure. Thermal injury is another complication that can be avoided by not using plaster larger than 10 ply and not using water hotter than 24°C.

Other complications that are less common, but may still arise, include cast saw cuts and burns if removal technique is insufficient, and thrombophlebitis, pulmonary embolus, or joint stiffness if utilized for excessive amounts of time.

VII. DELIVERING THE PATIENT TO POSTANESTHESIA UNIT

Following the procedure, patients will generally be awoken from anesthesia and extubated (if intubated for the procedure). At times, particularly in trauma cases, the patient may stay intubated or under induction of anesthesia. When transferring the patient from the OR table, make sure the stretcher is locked and staff are present on both sides of the table.

When a patient wakes up following surgery, he/she may be agitated and confused. It is appropriate to explain the surgery is complete and that you will be transferring them. Steps to ensure the patient's comfort and safe transfer include: Providing proper head elevation, anatomic positioning of the body and making sure all vital monitors are properly attached without any tangling of wires. In addition, set the IV on the stretcher and provide the appropriate amount of oxygen to the patient. Several techniques to ensure smooth transfer from the OR table to the stretcher or bed are available and include low-friction plastic bags, sleds, and "smooth movers."

During the transfer from the OR to the PACU, a member of both the surgical team and anesthesia team will physically transport the patient from the operating room to the postanesthesia unit. Here they will report to the appropriate station and provide the postanesthesia unit nurse with the relevant information related to the procedure and patient.

REFERENCES

1. Mathur P. Hand hygiene: back to the basics of infection control. *Indian J Med Res.* 2011;134(5):611-620.
2. Daniels JM. Introduction. In: Daniels MJ, Hoffman RM, eds. *Common Musculoskeletal Problems*. New York, NY: Springer International Publishing; 2015.
3. Roizen MF, Foss JF, Fischer SP. Preoperative evaluation. In: Miller RD, eds. *Anesthesia*. Philadelphia, PA: Churchill-Livingstone; 2000:824-883.
4. Boyce JM. Evidence in support of covering the hair of OR personnel. *AORN J.* 2014;99(1):4-8.
5. Noble WC. Dispersal of skin microorganisms. *Br J Dermatol.* 1975;93(4):477-485.
6. Shaw JA, Bordner MA, Hamory BH. Efficacy of the Steri-Shield filtered exhaust helmet in limiting bacterial counts in the operating room during total joint arthroplasty. *J Arthroplasty.* 1996;11(4):469-473.
7. Bliss MR, Thomas JM. Clinical trials with budgetary implications. Establishing randomised trials of pressure-relieving aids. *Prof Nurse.* 1993;8(5):292-296.
8. Conley DM, Singer SJ, Edmondson L, Berry WR, Gawande AA.. Effective surgical safety checklist implementation. *J Am Coll Surg.* 2011;212(5):873-879.
9. Hoppenfeld S, Buckley R. *Surgical Exposures in Orthopaedics: The Anatomic Approach*. Philadelphia, PA: Lippincott Williams & Wilkins, 2012.
10. Egol KA, Koval KJ, Zuckerman JD. *Handbook of Fractures*. Philadelphia, PA: Walters Kluwer, 2015.
11. Hemani ML, Lepor H. Skin preparation for the prevention of surgical site infection: which agent is best? *Rev Urol.* 2009;11(4):190-195.
12. Rynders SD, Hart J. *Orthopaedics for Physician Assistants*. Philadelphia, PA: Elsevier Health Sciences; 2013.

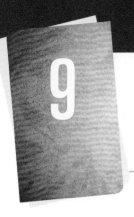

9

ADMINISTRATIVE SERVICES

Monica Racanelli

I. SUPPORTIVE SERVICES

The treatment and care of patients do not cease at the time they are discharged from the hospital. The support a patient receives postoperatively is critical to their ultimate outcome. Making arrangements for such supportive services is an important component of patient care. There are many home nursing care agencies in the United States. They provide a wealth of services to orthopaedic patients, including skilled nursing care, rehabilitation, personal care, and social work.

Skilled Nursing Care

- Injections: A skilled nursing staff can help with administration of injectable anticoagulants and offer training for patients and their caregivers.
- Wound Care: A wound care clinical nurse specialist can be arranged to provide in-home wound care for patients with slow-healing surgical wounds. For patients that are discharged from the hospital with negative pressure wound therapy systems (VAC), the wound care nurse specialist will provide appropriate VAC dressing changes and will often work in close collaboration with the provider. The VNS nurse may take digital photographs of the wound and securely e-mail them to the health care provider.
- Administering Medications: This service is especially useful for patients that require postoperative antibiotics via PICC line.

- Obtaining Labs: Patients receiving antibiotics often require frequent labs to monitor drug levels and inflammatory markers. These labs can be drawn at home and the results can be sent to the provider.
- Monitoring Vital Signs: Clinical measurements are taken to monitor temperature, blood pressure, pulse, and respiration rate.

In-Home Rehabilitation

- Physical Therapy: Physical therapists help restore strength, flexibility, coordination, and general function, all while patients remain at home in safe, comfortable, and familiar surroundings. The therapists follow a plan of care established by the physician and provide updates of changes in the patient's condition. These services are especially important for patients with joint replacements and those with fractures that have various comorbidities that make it difficult to get to an outpatient therapy location. Several studies have found that patients who followed acute hospital care with home care achieved clinical outcomes and quality of life scores that were similar or better than those who went to inpatient rehab facilities.[1,2]
- Occupational Therapy: Occupational therapists work with the patient to identify and eliminate environmental barriers and enhance participation in activities of daily living. They focus on enhancing fine motor skills, modifying tasks, and adapting the environment. They develop a specialized plan to meet the individual patient's need and work closely with the physical therapist and nursing staff.

Personal Care

- Cooking
- Bathing
- Grooming
- Laundry

- Housekeeping
- Shopping/Errands
- Companionship
- Escorting to and from doctor's visits.

Social Work

- Patient Care Coordination: The social worker helps coordinate the patient's care with all members of the home health care team to ensure a safe and timely discharge of home care. Such coordinated care and in-home services improve patients' overall compliance with the designed treatment plan.
- Supportive Counseling for Patients: A skilled social worker can provide the patient with guidance to enhance coping skills, reduce stress, and improve overall outlook.
- Caregiver Support: Social workers can provide the patient's family members with resources to help prevent burnout, strengthen coping skills, and increase the family's support systems.

II. THE FAMILY MEDICAL LEAVE ACT

The Family Medical Leave Act is a federal law that provides eligible employees up to 12 work weeks of unpaid, job-protected leave in a 12-month period. It requires employers to maintain group health benefits for the employee during this leave.[3] The FMLA also grants special provisions for military families, which include 26 weeks of FMLA leave in a single 12-month period to care for service member with a serious injury or illness.[4] The orthopaedic conditions that qualify for FMLA leave include:

- *Conditions that incapacitate the employee or a family member for more than three consecutive days.* The patient may receive ongoing treatment during this time, including appointments with health care provider, physical therapy, pain management, etc.

- *Conditions that require an overnight stay in a hospital or medical facility.* This includes multitrauma patients that require hospitalization, patients in rehabilitation institutions, and employees that require inpatient surgery.
- *Chronic conditions that cause occasional periods of incapacity and require treatment by health care provider at least twice a year.* For example, this may include patients with degenerative joint disease that requires periodic cortisone injections or patients with delayed union of fracture that require periodic radiographic evaluation.

There are several eligible reasons for employees to seek FMLA protection. In the specialty of Orthopaedics, there are typically three common reasons your patients may ask you to complete an FMLA form:

1. The first and most common reason you will be asked to complete an FMLA form is when a patient needs to take a medical leave and is unable to work owing to his **own FMLA-qualifying serious health condition**. This leave can be taken as an incapacity for a single continuous period of time, or the patient may choose to work part-time or on a reduced schedule while attending follow-up treatment appointments. There are several occupations that accommodate their employees with light duty or allow a reduced work schedule. This is an important discussion to have with the patient prior to completing the FMLA form.
2. The second reason you may encounter the FMLA form in your practice is for **an immediate family member of the patient** you are treating. The FMLA allows eligible employees to take a leave of absence to care for a relative with a serious health condition. Under FMLA, the definition of a relative is generally limited to a spouse, daughter, son, parent, and under certain circumstances, a sibling. A parent "in-law" is not a qualifying relative.
3. The third reason you may be asked to complete an FMLA form is for **intermittent leave**, which allows the patient to take a medical leave in separate blocks of time for a single qualifying

medical condition. This is often completed for patients with chronic, ongoing medical conditions. For example, a patient with degenerative joint disease of the knee may have episodic flare-up preventing him or her from performing their job functions. The patient may need to take a day or two off from work to rest, ice, and elevate their lower extremity. In this case, an FMLA form would be completed specifically for intermittent leave and it would provide FMLA protection for 12 months period.

III. WORKER'S COMPENSATION AND NO FAULT INSURANCE

Worker's Compensation is an insurance that provides cash benefits and medical care for workers who are injured as a direct result of their job. Employers pay for this insurance. The employer's insurance carrier will pay weekly cash benefits and provide medical care for the injured worker. In a Worker's Compensation case, no one party is designated to be at fault. A claim is paid to the injured worker if the employer or insurance carrier agrees that the injury is work related. If the employer or insurance carrier dispute the claim, a Worker's Compensation Board judge will decide who is right. The Worker's Compensation Board is a state agency that processes the claims and will determine whether the insurer will reimburse for cash benefits and medical care and the amounts payable.

Documentation

Proper documentation in the office note is essential when dealing with patients with worker's compensation insurance. Although the office visit forms and billing process may vary by state, there are generally four questions that need to be addressed by the provider in patient's office note at every visit:

1. Was the incident that the patient described the competent medical cause of the injury?

2. Are the patient's complaints and objective findings consistent with his/her history of injury?
3. Has the patient reached maximal medical improvement (MMI)?
4. What is the current level of disability/impairment?

Although the terminology may vary by state, in general, there are four categories of disability:

1. Temporary partial disability (Example: The patient is working reduced hours or light duty while recovering from injury.)
2. Temporary total disability (Example: The patient is unable to return to work for a temporary time period owing to work-related injury.)
3. Permanent partial disability (Example: The patient has a permanent impairment, but is able to return to work in some capacity.)
4. Permanent total disability (Example: The patient has a severe permanent impairment and will not be able to return to work in any capacity.)

Tip: These questions can be easily addressed by creating a WC template in your electronic medical record. The template can be inserted in the office note for patients with worker's compensation insurance. Here is a sample template:

"The work-related incident the patient described is the competent medical cause of this injury. Patient's complaints are consistent with the history of the injury. Patient's history of injury is consistent with the objective findings. There was no pre-existing condition. He/she has not yet reached maximal medical improvement. His/her current disability status is _____."

Prior Authorizations

Every state has different laws regarding Worker's Compensation prior authorizations. Several states require the physician to obtain prior authorization for surgical procedures, physical therapy, and specialist consultations. The requirements and process of prior authorization may vary from state to state. For instance, in

New York State, as of July 11, 2007, special diagnostic tests such as MRIs and CT scans that cost more than $1,000 require prior authorization. Prior authorization is not required for studies that cost less than $1,000.[5] If prior authorization is required in your state, be sure to request the service on the correct form. For example, in New York State, diagnostic services are requested on a C-4 Auth Form, whereas treatment such as hyperbaric oxygen therapy or acupuncture must be requested on MG-2 form. The health care provider's familiarize themselves with the worker's compensation process and commonly required forms in their state. Once the request is submitted, the insurance carrier typically has 30 days to respond to a request. During this period, the carrier may obtain an IME or records review. In order to deny a preauthorization request, the carrier must show a conflicting medical opinion.

Tip: When requesting authorization for a service or procedure, be sure to address that the need for the service/procedure is a result of the injury the patient sustained at work. Sample:

"Please take this letter as request for authorization of _____. The need for this study is a direct result of the injury the patient sustained at work on _____."

Independent Medical Examination

An Independent Medical Examination (IME) is a second opinion examination. The worker's compensation insurer may request an IME prior to giving authorization. The IME is a medical examination conducted by a health care provider chosen by and paid for by the insurer. If the physician performing the IME concludes that the patient's medical condition is not related to a work-related event or if the requested surgery or diagnostic study is not deemed medically necessary, the insurer may deny the claim or refuse to give authorization. Thus, the IME can have a large impact on the patient's case. However, an IME can be disputed by the patient as their attorney may request a hearing with a Worker's Compensation Judge to further discuss the case.

Final Impairment Rating

Once the patient reaches MMI, the medical provider is asked to assign an impairment rating. MMI is reached when a patient has recovered from the work-related injury to the greatest extent that is expected and no further improvement or deterioration in his or her condition is reasonably expected. When MMI has been reached, the physician must determine if the patient's injuries have lead to permanent impairment. If so, the patient can be assigned an impairment rating based on state laws. In 42 states, the medical provider will refer to one of the various editions of AMA Guide of Evaluation of Permanent Impairment. The other eight states—Florida, Illinois, Minnesota, New York, North Carolina, Oregon, Utah, and Wisconsin—provide their own state-specific guides for assigning an impairment rating. The compensation for permanent impairment is established by the statutes of each state. In most states, the worker's compensation guidelines provide a table, also referred to as a "schedule," to determine permanent impairment. Schedule loss of use awards are typically given for permanent impairment of extremities, loss of hearing, loss of vision, and facial disfigurement, whereas non-schedule permanent partial disability evaluations address impairments that were not amenable to schedule and include spine, pelvis, respiratory, cardiovascular, skin, and brain. In general, most orthopaedic injuries are amenable to schedule loss of use, which accounts for the severity of injury, loss of motion, and fracture type.[6]

No-fault Insurance

No-fault insurance, also called personal injury protection (PIP) insurance, is a type of automobile liability insurance that allows the policyholder to recover financial losses from the insurance company, regardless of who is at fault. There are currently twelve states and Puerto Rico that provide no-fault coverage. The states are Florida, Hawaii, Kansas, Kentucky, Massachusetts, Michigan, Minnesota, North Dakota, New Jersey, New York, Pennsylvania, and Utah.[7] Every state's no-fault laws and forms are different. The following are common New York State no-fault forms one may encounter:

- **NF-AOB**: No-Fault Assignment of Benefits (AOB) form is a legal contract in which the treating physician assumes the benefits of the personal injury protection portion of patients' automobile policy. If a patient wishes to receive medical treatment from a physician for injury sustained in an automobile accident, he or she must complete an AOB. This form is completed by the patient and typically submitted by the billing office.
- **NF-2:** In order to qualify for no-fault benefits, the patient must complete a no-fault application form (NF-2). This form must be filed within 30 days of the accident. Treating physicians are often required to produce proof that the NF-2 application was filed by the patient in a timely manner. If the NF-2 is not filed properly, the insurance carrier may not pay the bill.
- **NF-3**: This is a common form you will be required to complete as a health care provider treating patients with no-fault insurance. All no-fault medical treatment bills must be submitted on the "NF-3" form (No-Fault Verification of Treatment Form). This is an important form that the health care providers must complete and submit within 45 days from the date of treatment in order to get reimbursed for their services. The form includes basic patient demographic information, diagnosis, date of the patient's initial visit, disability status, need for physical therapy, and estimated duration of treatment. It also requires report of services rendered, which include date of service, place of service, description of treatment, and charges. This can be attached separately by the billing department.

IV. HANDICAP ALLOWANCES

Disabled Parking Permits

Reserved parking spaces are a legal requirement mandated by the ADA (Americans with Disabilities Act) for people with disabilities. Orthopaedic impairments are a common cause of physical disabilities. Consequently, one may frequently encounter applications for disabled parking permits in their practice. Disabled parking permits typically come in two forms:

1. Disabled parking placard/hangtag:
   - Offered for individuals with temporary or permanent disabilities.
2. Disabled license plate:
   - Reserved for individuals with permanent disabilities.

Temporary Parking Permit

- Typically valid for 6 months (up to 12 months in some states).
- Issued to a person with a temporarily disabling condition.
- The disabling condition must be one that limits a person's ability to ambulate temporarily and requires the use of an assistive device such as a cane, crutches, brace, walker, etc.

   Example: Ankle fracture, tibia fracture, femur fracture, lower extremity injury/surgery, spine injury/surgery, etc.

Permanent Parking Permit

- Typically valid for anywhere from 2 to 6 years, depending on the state.
- Generally requires additional forms and documentation from the physician.
- Issued to a person with a permanent condition that limits or impairs a person's mobility on a long-term basis and is not expected to change even with additional treatment.

   Example: Amputation, degenerative joint disease, congenital anomaly, neuromotor dysfunction, chronic conditions, etc.

Qualifying Conditions for Disabled Parking Permits

The medical requirements to qualify for a disabled parking permit vary from state to state. In general, a qualifying disability is one or more of the following impairments[8]:

- Inability to walk 200 ft. or more without stopping to rest.
- Inability to walk without the use of or assistance from any of the following: another person, brace, cane, crutch, prosthetic device, wheelchair, or other assistive device.
- Severely limited ability to walk owing to a neurologic, arthritic, or other orthopaedic condition.
- Neuromuscular dysfunction that severely impairs the ability to ambulate.
- Limited use, or no use, of one or both legs.
- Use of portable oxygen.
- A class III or IV cardiac condition in accordance with the American Heart Association standards.
- Restrictions as a result of lung disease.
- Legal blindness.
- Mental or developmental disorder.

Tips for Handling Parking Permit Applications

- For temporary parking permit applications, indicate that the patient requires the use of an assistive device and specify this assistive device (cane, crutch, wheelchair, etc.).
- For permanent parking applications, indicate how the patient's physical disability makes the use of public transportation difficult and requires the use of a private vehicle for transportation.
- Use terminology that is easily recognized by the Department of Motor Vehicles such as "severe mobility impairment."
- Disabled parking permits are an important privilege granted exclusively to those with qualifying disabilities. Learn the disabled parking permit laws and requirements for your state. Consider the patient's orthopaedic impairment carefully to determine if it warrants a disabled parking permit and qualifies under the jurisdiction's requirements. Health care providers are expected to avoid abuse of disabled parking permits.

V. PRIOR AUTHORIZATION

Prior Authorization is a process used by health insurance companies to determine if a prescribed medication, diagnostic imaging, procedure, or equipment is covered by the patient's health plan. This process was created to ensure that the prescribed service, medication, or equipment is appropriate, safe, medically necessary, and cost-effective. It is also known as prior approval, pre-authorization, pre-certification or notification.

How Do I Know If a Prescribed Medication or Health care Service Requires Prior Authorization?

1. For medications, you will often be alerted by the pharmacist when a prior authorization is required.
2. You may contact the patient's insurance company to find out if they require prior authorization for the prescribed health care service or medication.
3. You may check the insurance company's website to determine if prior authorization is required.

How Do I Obtain a Prior Authorization?

The process of obtaining prior authorization varies from insurer to insurer. Typically, there are three ways to obtain prior authorization:

1. You may obtain an electronic prior authorization online. This is generally the most efficient, time-saving method.
2. You may obtain prior authorization over the telephone by contacting the insurance company's prior authorization representative.
3. Some companies require completion and faxing of a prior authorization form. Having these readily available in the office will help streamline this process. Although most companies will respond in 1 to 2 days, some insurers may take longer.

Once Prior Authorization Has Been Requested, What Possible Decisions Can the Health Insurance Company Arrive at?

1. **Approved.** Once prior authorization is approved, the patient can fill his prescription or obtain the prescribed service.

2. Denied. If a prior authorization is denied, the insurance company will send you a letter regarding the reason for the adverse determination and an explanation of the appeal process. You may choose to appeal the decision and initiate a peer-to-peer review request. (See section on peer-to-peer reviews for details.)

3. **Additional information requested.** This response is typically received when an insurance company is missing some information prior to providing authorization. It is not a denial. This may be the result of a simple clerical error such as an incorrect CPT code or failing to note the location of the requested service.

4. **Step therapy is required.** Step therapy is a type of a prior authorization required by some insurance companies. Step therapy demands that patients try a medication or service preferred by the insurance provider first. This is known as "step one," which is usually a less expensive drug or test. If the patient shows an unsuccessful result from step one, then a more expensive drug or study, known as "step two," can be approved. You may request an exception to step therapy if your patient has already tried and failed a more affordable medication/study, or if you believe the prescribed medication/study is medically necessary.

Tips for Successfully Handling Prior Authorization

- Using the insurance company's website to obtain prior authorization typically generates a quicker response.
- Familiarize yourself with common health insurance companies' formularies. This will avoid the need for unnecessary prior authorizations.

- When possible, start patients on the generic form of a medication in the same therapeutic class.
- Every insurance company has its own list of medications that require prior authorization before they are covered. Get to know the drugs that are prescribed often in your practice that require prior authorization. Osteoporosis drugs, anabolic steroids, growth hormones, and fentanyl products are often on this list. Such lists are generally available on the health insurance company website.
- Pharmaceutical representatives can often assist in obtaining prior approval for medications such as Teriparatide (Forteo) or medical equipment such as bone stimulators. They will generally handle the paperwork required to obtain prior authorization once they have the necessary medical information.
- Health insurance companies have their own criteria that need to be met in order to obtain prior authorizations for certain diagnostic tests. For example, certain diagnoses require 6 weeks of conservative management, including nonsteroidal anti-inflammatory drugs (NSAIDs) and physical therapy, before an MRI can be approved. Be sure to follow the recommended treatment guidelines prior to ordering costly tests.
- Be sure to justify the need for the prescribed medication or study in your office note. A thorough medical note will enable your staff to provide the insurance company with the necessary medical information required to fulfill their criteria for providing prior authorization.

VI. PEER-TO-PEER REVIEW

A medical peer-to-peer review is a process offered by several insurance companies when an adverse determination has been made. This is generally a phone conversation between the patient's health care provider and a physician at the insurance company. It allows the patient's health care provider to challenge the adverse determination and offer additional information to a physician from the insurance company for reconsideration.

Tips for Handling a Peer-To-Peer Review

- Review the notice of denial from the insurance company prior to engaging in a peer-to-peer review. This letter will include the clinical rationale for the denial and information regarding the appeal process. Carefully reviewing the reason for denial will enable you to formulate your case to obtain approval.

- Confirm that the medication or test you ordered is in fact the one being denied. Submission of an erroneous CPT code is a common reason for denial.

- Review the insurance company's medical guidelines for the requested service. This will help you prove that your case does meet the insurance guidelines and was incorrectly rejected. If you find that the requested service is outside of the insurance guidelines, be prepared to provide peer-reviewed medical literature that supports the requested service.

- Have the patient's medical records available when making the peer-to-peer phone call. This will help you answer questions quickly and accurately.

- Schedule the peer-to-peer phone call at a time when you will be readily available. Inform your staff when you are expecting a peer-to-peer phone call. There is a limited period of time in which a peer-to-peer can be conducted.

- Be prepared to summarize your case with a brief history of present illness, current symptoms, pertinent physical examination, work-up performed so far, previous treatments and response to those treatments, current diagnosis, and your plan. Be concise and provide facts, not opinions.

VII. NARCOTIC PRESCRIPTIONS

The Drug Enforcement Administration (DEA) is the primary federal agency responsible for enforcing the Controlled Substance Act (CSA). This dictates the federal law regarding both illicit and licit controlled substances. In order to prescribe controlled substances, practitioners must register with the DEA and obtain a license number. The drugs and other products that are considered control substances are divided into five schedules (Table 9-1). The DEA laws for practitioners vary from state to state and should be reviewed regularly.[9]

Tips on Prescribing Narcotic Pain Medications

- Clarify the appropriate dosage, frequency, and side effects of the medication with the patient. Discuss the maximum daily dosage.
- Some patients are prone to constipation with use of narcotics. Prescribe stool softener, if needed.
- Inform the patient that opioids are intended for short-term pain relief. Unless contraindicated, substitute NSAIDs for breakthrough pain and to minimize the need for opioids.
- Stress the importance of modalities that may alleviate pain. Cryotherapy has been shown to decrease pain and narcotic medication requirement during the first 24 postoperative hours.[10]
- Opioid dependence and overdose has become a significant public health issue in the United States. Educate the patient about the risk of dependence and addiction and encourage the patient to discontinue the narcotics as soon as the pain improves.
- If the patient exhibits signs of narcotic abuse or addiction, inform your supervising physician and discuss referral to pain management specialist.

TABLE 9-1	DEA Drug Schedules
Description	**Examples**
Schedule I	
The substances in the schedule have not currently been accepted for medical use in the United States, lack accepted safety for use under medical supervision, and have a high potential for abuse.	Heroin, Lysergic Acid Diethylamide (LSD), Peyote, Methylene-dimethoxy-methamphetamine ("ecstasy") Note: Currently, marijuana remains in the schedule I category despite the calls for reclassification. There are several studies underway to address the safety and efficacy of marijuana.
Schedule II, IIN	
The substances and the schedule have a high potential for abuse with severe psychological and physical dependence. These drugs include certain narcotics, depressants, and stimulants.	Schedule II: Hydrocodone, Oxycodone, Hydromorphone, Fentanyl, Methadone, Morphine, Opium, Pantopon, and Meperidine. Schedule IIN: Non-narcotics such as Amphetamine, Methamphetamine, and Nabilone
Schedule III, IIIN	
Substances in this schedule have less potential of abuse than substances in Schedules I or II. Abuse of these drugs may lead to moderate to low physical or psychological dependence.	Schedule III: Products containing not more than 90 mg of codeine per dosage unit (Tylenol with Codeine), and buprenorphine. Schedule IIIN: Non-narcotics such as benzphetamine, phendimetrazine, ketamine, testosterone, and anabolic steroids.

(*continued*)

TABLE 9-1

DEA Drug Schedules (*continued*)

Schedule IV	
Substances in this schedule have a low potential for abuse and low risk of abuse relative to substances in Schedule III.	Alprazolam, carisoprodol, clonazepam, diazepam, lorazepam, midazolam, temazepam, and triazolam.
Schedule V	
Substances in this schedule have a low potential for abuse relative to substances in Schedule IV. This schedule consist of preparations containing limited quantities of certain narcotics.	Cough preparations containing not more than 200 mg of codeine per 100 mL or per 100 g (Robitussin AC, Phenergan with Codeine), and ezogabine.

REFERENCES

1. Mallinson TR, Bateman J, Tseng H-Y, et al. A comparison of discharge functional status after rehabilitation in skilled nursing, home health, and medical rehabilitation settings for patients after lower-extremity joint replacement surgery. *Arch Phys Med Rehabil.* 2011;92:712-720.
2. Mahomed NN, Davis AM, Hawker G, et al. Inpatient compared with home-based rehabilitation following primary unilateral total hip or knee replacement: a randomized controlled trial. *J Bone Joint Surg Am.* 2008;90(8):1673-1680.
3. Fact Sheet #28A: Employee Protections under the FMLA. September, 2012. https://www.dol.gov/whd/regs/compliance/whdfs28a.pdf. Accessed June 15, 2017.
4. Fact Sheet #28M: The Military Leave Provisions under the FMLA. February, 2013. https://www.dol.gov/whd/regs/compliance/whdfs28m.pdf. Accessed June 15, 2017.
5. Increase in Medical Authorization Request Threshold. June, 2007. http://www.wcb.ny.gov/content/main/SubjectNos/sn046_197.jsp. Accessed June 15, 2017.

6. New York State Guidelines for Determining Permanent Impairment and Loss of Wage Earning Capacity. December, 2012. http://www.wcb.ny.gov/content/main/hcpp/ImpairmentGuidelines/2012ImpairmentGuide.pdf. Accessed June 15, 2017.

7. No-Fault Auto Insurance. III. February, 2014. http://www.iii.org/issue-update/no-fault-auto-insurance. Accessed June 15, 2017.

8. Application for Parking Permit or License Plate, for Persons with Severe Disabilities. NYS-DMV. April, 2016. https://dmv.ny.gov/forms/mv6641.pdf. Accessed June 15, 2017.

9. Mid-Level Practitioners Authorization by State. DEA. September, 2016. https://www.deadiversion.usdoj.gov/drugreg/practioners/mlp_by_state.pdf. Accessed June 15, 2017.

10. Osbahr DC, Cawley PW, Speer KP. The effect of continuous cryotherapy on glenohumeral joint and subacromial space temperatures in the postoperative shoulder. *Arthroscopy*. 2002; 18(7):748-754.

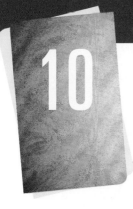

TIPS AND TRICKS OF THE TRADE

Monica Racanelli

I. MEDICAL SUPPLIES

- Arm Sling (Figure 10-1)
  - Indications: Minimally displaced clavicle fractures, proximal humerus fractures, immobilization after shoulder dislocations, strains, and postoperative immobilization after upper extremity surgery.
  - Application: Position the elbow in the pocket of the sling. Place the strap over opposite shoulder, feed through the D-ring, and secure to itself. Hand should be elevated slightly above the elbow when secured. Many different variations of the arm sling are available in the market.
  - Advantages: Easy to use. Provides proper immobilization and support of the shoulder and elbow joints.
  - Disadvantages: Can cause discomfort and skin irritation.
- Sarmiento Brace (Figure 10-2)
  - Indications: Closed humeral shaft fractures in acceptable alignment. Acceptable alignment of humeral shaft fracture is considered to be:
    - 20 degrees anterior/posterior angulation
    - 30 degrees of varus/valgus angulation
    - Up to 3 cm of shortening
  - Application: The brace consists of 2 shells applied either anterior–posterior or medial–lateral, and secured with Velcro straps. Use a collar and cuff to support the forearm. Provide additional padding around the collar to reduce discomfort

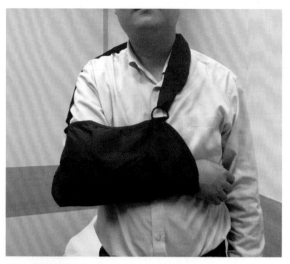

Figure 10-1 **Arm sling.** Proper placement of arm sling.

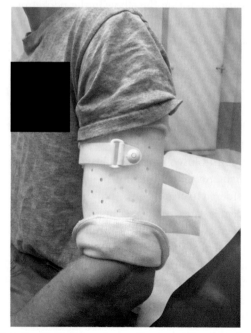

Figure 10-2 **Sarmiento brace.** Proper placement of Sarmiento Brace.

and avoid skin irritation. Avoid the use of a standard sling, which could cause fracture angulation.

■ Advantages: The fracture alignment is maintained through soft-tissue compression and gravity assistance. The brace permits early motion of the adjacent joints, giving providers the opportunity to encourage patients to begin early range-of-motion (ROM) exercises of the finger, wrist, elbow, and shoulder as tolerated.

■ Disadvantages: Contraindicated in patients with massive soft-tissue injury. Requires close supervision and follow-up with radiographs to ensure maintenance of reduction. Frequent brace adjustments are needed as swelling subsides.

■ Hinged Elbow Brace (Figure 10-3)

■ Indications: Elbow instability, dislocation, collateral ligament repair or biceps/triceps repair. Also applicable in postsurgery or postinjury patients who have regained inadequate motion.

■ Application: Adjust the brace to fit the patient's arm. Apply the brace, fasten the straps, and adjust the ROM dial as needed.

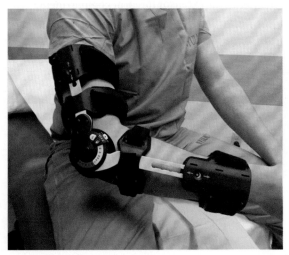

Figure 10-3 **Hinged elbow brace.** Proper placement of hinged elbow brace.

- Advantages: Allows for early, protected ROM, permitting extension and flexion while reducing varus and valgus stress. Hinges can be adjusted weekly to allow for improvement in elbow ROM.
- Disadvantages: Must be applied properly to be effective.
- Static-Progressive Splints
  - Indications: Used to gain ROM in patients with joint stiffness. It is typically used as an additional modality in patients who have regained inadequate motion with standard therapy or have plateaued in therapy.
  - Application: Similar to hinged elbow brace.
  - Advantages: Allows for improvements in elbow ROM.
  - Disadvantages: May cause discomfort.
  - Note: When ordering the splint, specify the joint and function, that is, static-progressive supination/pronation forearm splint.
- Counterforce Tennis Elbow Strap (Figure 10-4)
  - Indication: Lateral epicondylitis.
  - Application: Wrap around the forearm, approximately 2.5 cm distal to the lateral epicondyle. Some straps have additional gel pads or pillows which should be placed against the radial muscles of the extensor forearm compartment.

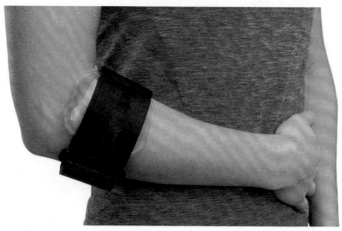

Figure 10-4 **Tennis elbow strap.** Proper placement of tennis elbow strap.

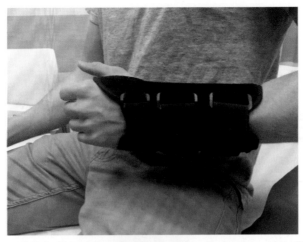

Figure 10-5 **Cock-up wrist splint.** Proper placement of cock-up wrist splint.

- Advantages: The strap is thought to decrease the pressure on extensor carpi radialis brevis tendon by dispersing the muscle contraction forces. It is inexpensive, adjustable, and easy to fit.
- Disadvantages: Improper use can lead to nerve irritation.
- Cock-up wrist splint (Figure 10-5)
    - Indications: Carpal tunnel syndrome, wrist sprain or tendinitis, buckle fracture, post-wrist or hand surgery.
    - Application: This is a removable wrist orthosis that can be applied and secured with Velcro straps. It typically contains a metal or thermoplastic insert in its volar (or dorsal) compartment providing rigid support.
    - Advantages: Provides wrist stability/immobilization, while allowing digital motion and forearm rotation. Easy to use and cost-effective.
    - Disadvantages: More rigid and less comfortable than custom-made thermoplastic splints.
- Hinged knee brace (Figure 10-6)
    - Indications: MCL or LCL tear, MCL or LCL repair, post-op use after knee surgery to prevent valgus and varus stress.

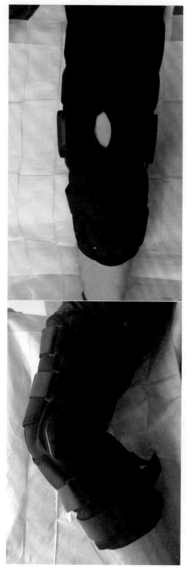

Figure 10-6 **Hinged knee brace.** Proper placement of hinged knee brace.

- ▪ Application: Adjust the brace to fit the patient's leg. When applying the brace, be sure to align the hinges around the medial and lateral aspect of the knee. Fasten the straps and adjust the ROM dial as needed.
- ▪ Advantages: Hinges can be adjusted to allow for advancement in ROM. Protects against varus and valgus stress.
- ▪ Disadvantages: Must be applied properly to be effective.
- ▪ Custom-made Functional ACL Brace
    - ▪ Indications: ACL or PCL instability, ACL or PCL reconstruction, prophylactic use (controversial).
    - ▪ Application: The brace must be ordered through a local distributor. Measurements are obtained using anatomic reference points and the brace is custom-made to fit the patient. The brace reduces knee translation and rotation.
    - ▪ Advantages: Because it is custom-made, it can accommodate a broad spectrum of knee sizes. It can be customized with a variety of options and accessories. It has been reported to subjectively improve stability and function and can be used as an adjunct to graft protection after ACL reconstruction.[1,2]
    - ▪ Disadvantages: Expensive. It can require multiple trips to the orthotist for proper fitting. It can increase energy expenditure and decrease agility.[3,4] Relative lack of conclusive research on prophylactic benefits. Brace effectiveness diminishes at physiologic stress levels.[5,6]
- ▪ Patellofemoral brace ("J" brace, Palumbo brace) (Figure 10-7)
    - ▪ Indications: Patellofemoral syndrome, patellar subluxation or dislocation, patellar tendinitis, post-op management (lateral release).
    - ▪ Application: Usually made from an elastic material such as neoprene and may include straps and buttresses to stabilize the patella. To apply, pull the brace onto affected leg and align patella in center of cutout. Secure the counterbalancing straps, if present, in moderate tension.
    - ▪ Advantages: Low cost, ease to use, widely available. Designed to improve patellar tracking with medially directed

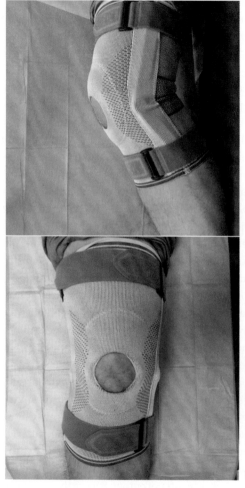

Figure 10-7 Palumbo brace. Proper placement of palumbo brace.

force.[7] Changes in regional temperature, neurosensory feedback, and circulation may also contribute to its effects.[8] Has been shown to improve anterior knee pain in several studies.[9,10]

- Disadvantages: Subjective benefits exceed objective findings. Some studies found the brace to be ineffective.[11,12] Can cause skin irritation.

- Knee Immobilizer (Figure 10-8)
  - Indications: Stabilization after acute knee injury, quadriceps or patellar tendon rupture, patellar fracture or dislocation, post-op immobilization.
  - Application: Consists of rigid struts, foam liner, and Velcro straps. To apply, open all the Velcro straps and liner, place behind the leg with the strut centered, wrap the foam liner around the leg and secure the Velcro straps.
  - Advantages: Inexpensive, widely available, easy to apply.
  - Disadvantages: Tends to slide down when ambulating, thus requiring frequent adjustments. Extended use may lead to knee stiffness and muscle atrophy.

- Unloader Knee Brace for Osteoarthritis (Figure 10-9)
  - Indications: Unicompartmental knee osteoarthritis, knee malalignment.
  - Application: Can be off-the-shelf or custom-made. Most braces use a three-point leverage design applying external varus or valgus force to the knee which distracts the involved compartment and reduces the load.[13-15]
  - Advantages: Shown to reduce pain, improve function, and reduce the use of pain meds in patients with unicompartmental OA.[14,16]
  - Disadvantages: Expensive. Brace efficacy depends on proper application. Low compliance rate due to brace discomfort, poor fit, and skin irritation.[17]

- CPM Machine (Figure 10-10)
  - Indications: Commonly used to maintain joint motion after knee manipulation and release of arthrofibrosis. May be used

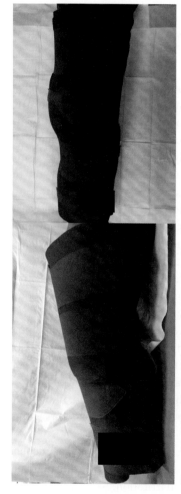

Figure 10-8 Knee immobilizer. Proper placement of knee immobilizer.

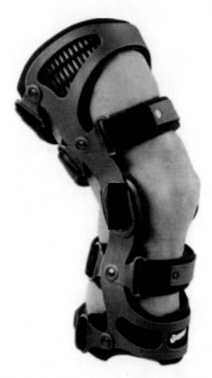

Figure 10-9 **Unloader brace.** Proper placement of unloader brace around knee.

after knee replacements, ACL reconstructions, microfracture, autologous chondrocyte transplantation, and chondroplasties.

- Application: Motorized device applied externally to enable the joint to move passively through a predetermined ROM. ROM, speed, and hold times can be altered as needed.
- Advantages: Helpful in maintaining ROM and reducing edema. Movement of synovial fluid allows for better diffusion of nutrients into damaged cartilage.[18,19]
- Disadvantages: Does not improve long-term knee function. Can be cumbersome and difficult for patients to use properly at home. Can cause increased discomfort. Some studies show no added benefit in functional recovery after TKR.[20]

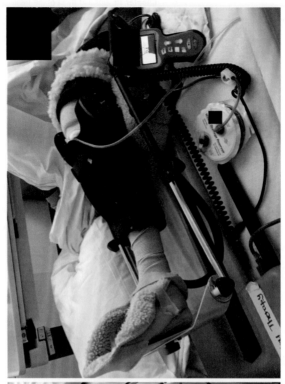

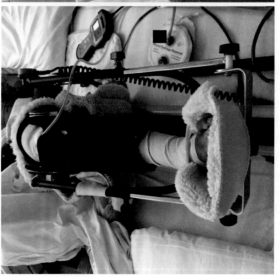

Figure 10-10 **CPM machine.** Proper patient positioning in CPM machine.

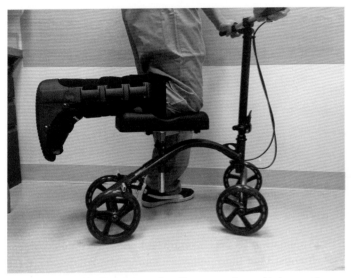

Figure 10-11 **Steerable knee walker.** Proper use of steerable knee walker.

- Steerable Knee Scooter (Roll-A-Bout walker) (Figure 10-11)
  - Indications: Also known as a knee walker, coaster, or cruiser. Any ankle or foot injury/surgery/condition that requires the patient to be nonweight bearing (NWB) on the lower extremity.
  - Application: A two-, three-, or four-wheeled device that has a knee pad to support the shin of the affected extremity. The opposite foot makes contact with the ground to provide propulsion.
  - Advantages: Excellent alternative to crutches. Allows patients to be NWB safely. Comfortable and easy to maneuver. Allows patients to be active and mobile during the rehabilitation period. Can be rented temporarily.
  - Disadvantages: Heavier and more difficult to load in a vehicle than crutches. Cannot negotiate stairs.
- Ankle Air-Stirrup brace (eg, Aircast) (Figure 10-12)
  - Indications: Acute ankle sprain.

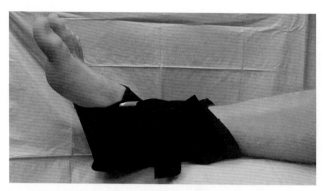

Figure 10-12 Aircast. Proper placement of Aircast.

- Application: This is a semi-rigid, functional ankle brace. It consists of thermoplastic countered medial and lateral shells lined with air-filled foam pads held together by encircling Velcro straps and adjustable heel pad. The air-filled pads provide support and graduated compression during ambulation to promote edema reduction. When applying the brace, adjust the heel attachment connecting the medial and lateral shell to ensure a snug fit. Apply the bottom encircling strap first, and then proceed to the top strap. The brace should be worn with socks and can fit inside most lace sneakers.
- Advantages: Provides ankle support, protection, and comfort. It allows dorsiflexion and plantarflexion of the ankle, while providing medial and lateral control. Can be worn inside most wide shoes or sneakers. Studies have shown that functional treatment of acute ankle sprains promotes better outcomes.[21]
- Disadvantages: The brace may loosen, slip, and require frequent adjustments.
- Lace-up ankle brace (Figure 10-13)
  - Indication: Acute and chronic ankle sprain/injury.

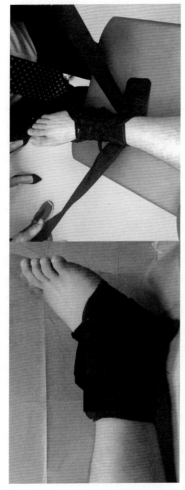

Figure 10-13 Lace-up ankle brace. Proper placement of lace-up ankle brace.

- Application: The material and design vary from brand to brand. This brace is low profile, typically consists of lace in the front of the foot, and stabilizing straps that are wrapped in a figure-of-eight fashion to provide additional subtalar joint support. Some braces have removable metal or plastic stays for added medial and lateral stability.
- Advantages: Easy to use, reusable, and adjustable. Easily fits inside most athletic shoes. External ankle support has been shown to improve proprioception.[22,23]
- Disadvantages: The effectiveness of the lace-up ankle brace is controversial, with studies revealing conflicting results. A common concern is that prolonged lace-up ankle brace may lead to ankle weakness, which would consequently make the ankle prone to injury.
- Arizona brace (Figure 10-14)
  - Indication: Designed for treatment of posterior tibialis tendon dysfunction (PTTD).
  - Application: This is a custom-fabricated orthoses typically made from leather and thermoplastic. It holds the foot in a neutral position and out of valgus by using a three-point fixation similar to a well-molded cast. It requires custom casting and fitting and is designed to fit inside a comfort shoe.
  - Advantages: The Arizona brace is clinically proven to be effective at treating Stage I and II PTTD. It has been shown to improve clinical symptoms, ankle and foot alignment, and functional outcomes in patients with PTTD, with success rates up to 90%.[24-27]
  - Disadvantages: The Arizona brace relies on passively correcting the deformity, thus the results are less favorable in patients with Stage III PTTD.
- Ankle–Foot Orthoses (AFO) (Figure 10-15)
  - Indication: Mainly used to correct foot drop.
  - The AFOs are classified into four major categories[28,29]:
    - *Flexible AFO*: Provides dorsiflexion assistance, but poor stabilization of subtalar joint.

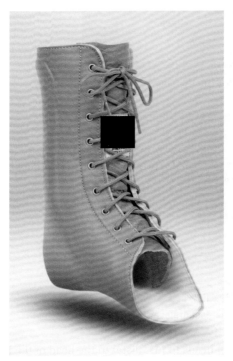

Figure 10-14 **Arizona brace.** Depiction of Arizona brace.

- *Rigid AFO*: Blocks ankle motion and stabilizes the subtalar joint. Provides possibility of controlling forefoot adduction and abduction.
- *Anti-Talus AFO*: Blocks ankle motion, especially dorsiflexion. Poor stabilization of subtalar joint.
- *Tamarack Flexure Joint AFO:* Provides subtalar stabilization, while allowing ankle dorsiflexion and plantar flexion. Some designs provide dorsiflexion assistance to correct foot drop.
- Application: AFO can be prefabricated or custom-made. It is generally constructed of lightweight polypropylene-based plastic in the shape of an "L," extending from distal to the

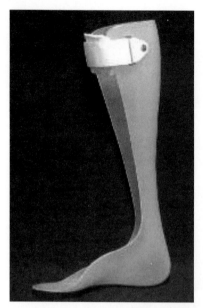

Figure 10-15 **Ankle–foot orthoses (AFO).** Depiction of AFO.

metatarsal heads to just distal to the head of the fibula. It attaches to the calf and foot with straps and fit inside most shoes. It can be rigid or come with ankle hinges.

- Advantages: AFOs are lightweight and help correct foot drop, limit the development of contractures, enable the foot to fit inside a shoe, and improve the ability to ambulate.
- Disadvantages: Immobilizing effect of the brace can cause ankle stiffness.

II. OTHER THERAPIES

Bone Growth Stimulators

Bone growth stimulators are promoted as safe, noninvasive devices that stimulate fracture healing. They are easy to use, painless, and have built-in software to track treatments. The bone stimulators generally used in Orthopaedics are classified into two groups:

electromagnetic and ultrasound. The electrical bone stimulator generates a low-level electrical field which activates the body's repair mechanism and promotes bone healing. Low-intensity pulsed ultrasound devices send ultrasound waves through the skin and soft tissue to the fracture, activating a biologic healing response at the molecular level.[30] The bone stimulators can be applied directly on the skin over the fracture site, over a cast, or can be incorporated in a cast. The efficacy and cost-effectiveness of bone growth stimulators on fracture healing remain inconclusive and controversial.

Platelet-Rich Plasma Therapy

Platelet-rich plasma (PRP) is blood plasma that is enriched with autologous platelets. It is theorized that the high concentration of certain growth factors and cytokines found within PRP stimulates healing of bone and soft tissue wherever they are applied. The platelets release proliferative and morphogenic proteins that work together to induce a healing response. There are a variety of PRP preparation systems available in the market that can be used in the office setting and the operating room. Each commercially marketed PRP system has its own preparation protocol. In general, the process of PRP therapy involves collecting the patient's whole blood by venipuncture that can be anticoagulated with citrate dextrose, followed by two-stage centrifugation to separate red blood cells and concentrate platelets. The PRP yield from venous blood draw may vary depending on patient's baseline platelet count, the device used, and the technique employed.[31] The effectiveness of PRP has yet to be definitively established, and thus its use is still somewhat controversial.

III. REHABILITATION PROTOCOLS

These rehabilitation guidelines can be altered based on individual patient's progress. Patients progress at different rates depending on their age, comorbidities, preinjury condition, severity of injury, tissue quality, and rehabilitation compliance. Rehabilitation protocols vary among physicians with regard to timing of progression and appropriate therapeutic exercise. Although rehabilitation protocols are generally based on scientific rationale, it is also influenced by the physician's clinical experience and expert opinion. Close communication with the physician is an essential component in designing an appropriate and effective rehabilitation program for the patient. This communication should continue throughout the recovery process and rehab instructions should be tailored to individual patients to ensure a successful outcome.

Patient education is an important component of the first postoperative visit. For example:

- Adjust the sling, if needed. Instruct the patient on how to don and doff sling safely and properly.
- Discuss the importance of cryotherapy in decreasing pain and swelling and minimizing the inflammatory process.
- When warranted, demonstrate to the patient how to perform pendulum exercises during the office visit and have the patient demonstrate the exercises to ensure proper technique.
- Pain associated with sleeping is a common complaint after shoulder surgery. Discuss sleeping postures and modification that may provide comfort. Suggest sleeping in a reclined position rather than lying flat on the back. Sleeping in a reclining chair is ideal for the first few weeks after surgery. If a recliner is not available, the patient may bolster himself from behind with pillows for comfort. A single pillow placed under the elbow and hand also puts the shoulder in a comfortable position while sleeping.
- Review the operative findings and precautions with the patient.

Clavicle Fracture ORIF

Therapy instructions may vary based on the severity of the clavicle fracture (degree of comminution), soft-tissue damage, and type of fixation. It is important to communicate with the surgeon to verify therapy instructions and tailor the rehab protocol accordingly. In general, therapy will begin with gentle motion exercises. Strengthening exercises will be added gradually as the fracture heals.

0 to 6 Weeks

- Sling application for comfort. Remove sling for ROM exercises.
- Ice application.
- Pendulum exercises.
- Gentle active range of motion (AROM)/passive range of motion (PROM) of the shoulder. Limit forward elevation to 90 degrees.
- Avoid overhead exercises.
- Avoid lifting more than 5 lb.
- AROM/PROM elbow, forearm, wrist, and hand. Cervical ROM exercises.
- Isometric R.C. stretching and strengthening.
- Soft-tissue treatment/modalities as needed.

6 to 12 Weeks

- Discontinue sling.
- AROM/PROM of shoulder, elbow, forearm, wrist, and hand as tolerated.
- Begin resistive R.C. stretching and strengthening.
- Scapular mobilization and stabilizer strengthening.
- Scar management.
- Modalities as needed.

Arthroscopic Rotator Cuff Repair

The rehabilitation program for rotator cuff repairs is tailored to each individual patient based on the size of tear, tendons involved, tissue quality, strength of repair, and concomitant procedures performed. These factors determine the pace at which a patient will progress through different phases of therapy and their ultimate outcome. Rehabilitation protocols for rotator cuff repairs are commonly divided into four phases, progressing from a protective phase and gradually moving to a strengthening phase.[32] Advancement to the next phase of rehabilitation depends on when the patient reaches the ROM goals and meets the established timelines. Rehabilitation protocols can vary between surgeons with respect to timing of progression and appropriate therapeutic exercises. Close communication with the surgeon and the physical therapist is imperative in order to design the optimal rehab protocol for the patient.

Phase I (0 to 6 Weeks)

Goal: During the first 6 weeks, there is increased collagen deposition and growth factors at the site of the repair, which should not be exposed to excessive stress. The goal in the first phase is to minimize stress placed on the repaired tissues, while maintaining shoulder ROM. Formal therapy is optional for the first 4 to 6 weeks. The patient may perform pendulum exercises at home three times per day.

- Sling application for 4 to 6 weeks. Remove sling for exercise and showers only.
- Cryotherapy/ice application.
- Begin pendulum exercises, 3 times per day.
- Gentle PROM right shoulder (therapist-assisted or self-assisted with use of nonoperative UE).
- If subscapularis tendon is repaired, passive external rotation should be restricted.
- Isolated scapular depression and protraction. (Avoid scapula retraction and scapula clock exercises due to increased stress on supraspinatus muscle.[33])
- AROM/PROM elbow, forearm, wrist, hand, and cervical spine.
- Avoid any AROM of the shoulder.
- Avoid lifting more than a coffee mug.
- Other modalities as needed.

Phase II (6 weeks to 3 months)

Goal: This is the remodeling phase. During this phase, gentle stress placed on the newly formed collagen matrix facilitates fiber orientation and enhancing tensile strength of the repair. The focus during this phase is to restore shoulder ROM, both passively and actively, while protecting the healing tissues.

- Discontinue sling.
- Begin active assisted range of motion (AAROM), followed by AROM of the shoulder.
- Continue PROM/pendulums of the shoulder as tolerated.
- Continue AROM/PROM elbow, forearm, wrist, hand, and cervical spine.
- Initiate neuromuscular control exercises.
- Work on scapulothoracic kinematics.
- Submaximal isometric external and internal rotation exercises.
- Open-chain proprioceptive activities.
- Continue ice application and other modalities as needed.

Phase III (3 to 6 months)

Goal: This is the rotator cuff strengthening phase. At this point, there should be sufficient tendon-to-bone healing to withstand gradual strengthening exercises. The objective of this phase is to improve strength and function through gradually progressed resistive exercises. The patient should gradually return to functional activities by the end of this phase.

- Continue AROM, AAROM, PROM of the shoulder.
- Begin gradual R.C. stretching and strengthening (Theraband exercise).
- Begin active stretching program for the shoulder.
- Periscapular strengthening.
- Scapular stabilization exercises.
- Isotonic shoulder exercises.
- Continue neuromuscular control and proprioceptive exercises.
- Closed chain stability exercises.
- Continue modalities as needed.

Phase IV (6 to 9 months)

Goal: This is the advanced strengthening phase. It is essentially a progression of the previous phase with a focus on sport-specific rehabilitation activities. At this juncture, the repaired rotator cuff tissue has matured enough to endure more stress than the previous phase. The goal of this phase is to increase strength and endurance and return to recreational sport activities.

- Continue all exercises from Phase III.
- Progressive strengthening of the rotator cuff.
- Advanced rhythmic stabilization exercises.
- Plyometrics of the upper extremity.
- Sport-specific training exercises.
- Maintenance exercise program for endurance and flexibility.

Proximal Humerus Fracture ORIF

Therapy instructions may vary based on type of fracture, type of fixation, and concomitant injuries. Isolated greater tuberosity fractures that are fixed with sutures may follow a rehabilitation protocol similar to rotator cuff repair. It is essential to communicate with the surgeon in order to design an appropriate and effective rehabilitation program for the individual patient.

- Sling application for comfort.
- Ice application.
- Pendulums.
- Begin PROM shoulder as tolerated.
- Begin AROM/AAROM (when cleared by physician).
- Begin R.C. stretching and strengthening (when cleared by physician).
- AROM/PROM elbow, forearm, wrist, hand, and cervical spine.
- Scar management.
- Modalities as needed.

Carpal Tunnel Syndrome

- Night-time cock-up wrist splint application $\times$ 6 weeks.
- Nerve gliding exercises.
- Isolated tendon gliding exercises.

- Modalities including ultrasound, fluidotherapy, and iontophoresis.
- Ergonomic education.

Trochanteric Bursitis

- Hip abductor stretching and strengthening (gluteus maximus, gluteus medius, gluteus minimus, tensor fascia lata)
- AROM/PROM hip.
- Modalities as needed.
- Home program.

Quadriceps or Patellar Tendon Rupture Repair

Precautions, ROM limits, and specific timeframes may be altered based on the integrity of the repair and associated injuries. Some patients with massive quadriceps tendon rupture repair may be placed in a cylinder cast keeping the knee in full extension of 4 weeks. Verify the rehabilitation instructions with surgeon for individual patients.

0 to 4 weeks

- Weight bearing as tolerated (WBAT) in knee immobilizer or hinged knee brace locked in full extension.
- Elevation and ice application.
- If ROM is allowed, patient may begin gentle active and active assisted knee flexion and passive knee extension. Limit ROM within 0 to 45 degrees (check with physician regarding ROM limits).
- Modalities as needed.

4 to 8 weeks

- WBAT in knee immobilizer or hinged knee brace locked in full extension. May begin weaning off brace at 6 weeks.
- AROM/PROM knee within 0 to 90 degrees with gradual progression (when cleared by physician).
- Begin isometric stretching and strengthening exercises (when cleared by physician).
- Patella mobilization.
- Modalities as needed.

8 to 12 weeks

- Discontinue brace.
- AROM/PROM knee as tolerated.
- Quad and hamstring strengthening.
- Proprioception exercises.
- Modalities as needed.

ACL Reconstruction

A well-designed rehabilitation protocol for ACL reconstruction is adapted to patient's specific needs and level of athletics. The protocol can be varied based on graft selection, patient population, and concomitant injuries. There are different phases of rehabilitation, and the progression from one phase to the next is generally based on the patient achieving functional criteria rather than time elapsed since surgery.[34] Consult the surgeon regarding progression of therapy and return to sport criteria of individual patients.

0 to 4 Weeks after Surgery

Goal: Control pain, decrease swelling, protect the graft, regain quadriceps control, restore full passive knee extension and gradually restore knee flexion, and restore normalized gait.

- Immediately post-op, patient may be WBAT in a locked knee brace in full extension, with the use of crutches. Brace should be unlocked at first post-op visit. Crutches may be discontinued when normal gait is achieved and patient is able to safely ascend/descend stairs.
- Elevation, cryotherapy, other modalities as needed.
- Isometric quad contraction with knee in full extension.
- Begin AROM/PROM knee as tolerated. Stress full knee extension.
- Begin closed chain kinetic exercises for quad strengthening (mini-squats, wall sits, leg press).
- Patella and soft-tissue mobilization.
- Calf raises.
- May begin stationary bike.

4 to 12 Weeks after Surgery

Goal: Achieve full ROM, improve lower extremity strength, achieve normal gait without brace or assistive device.

- Discontinue knee brace.
- Full AROM/PROM knee as tolerated.
- Continue closed chain kinetic exercises for hip, quad, hamstring, and calf strengthening.
- Proprioception exercises (provided adequate quad control).
- Begin cross-training machines (avoid varus and valgus deviations).
- Continue patella mobilization.

12 to 20 Weeks after Surgery

Goal: Regain dynamic stability, begin plyometric exercises, increase endurance and strength.

- Plyometrics program (box jumps, scissor jumps, single leg hops, tuck jumps, landing techniques).
- Pre-running drills (low skips, punch steps, huddle walks, kick-backs, step-overs).
- Advanced proprioceptive exercises/neuromuscular training (single-leg dynamic balance, dual task balance).
- May begin jogging straight ahead.
- Jumping rope.
- Lunges sideways/forward
- Graduated return to running (begin on treadmill and transition to level outdoor surface).

20 to 24 Weeks after Surgery

Goal: Gradual, progressive return to sports, begin agility drills, restore full function, improve endurance and strength.

- Sport-specific training drills and exercises.
- Agility drills (zig-zags, cutting, side shuffles).
- Reactive jumping.

- Interval training.
- Running on all levels.
- Continue strengthening while advancing resistance and repetitions.
- Continue plyometrics.

Tibial Plateau Fracture

0 to 6 weeks

- Patient is placed in a hinged knee brace, unlocked. Brace may be removed for showers and therapy.
- NWB on the affected lower extremity.
- Begin AROM/PROM knee.
- Isometric quad and hamstring stretching and strengthening.
- Avoid varus and valgus stress.
- Modalities as needed.

6 to 10 weeks

- Discontinue hinged knee brace.
- Remain NWB on affected lower extremity.
- Continue AROM/PROM knee.
- Quad and hamstring stretching and strengthening.
- Modalities as needed.

10 to 16 weeks

- Advance to WBAT when clinically and radiographically healed.
- Continue AROM/PROM knee.
- Advanced lower extremity stretching and strengthening.
- Modalities as needed.

Ankle Fracture ORIF

0 to 6 weeks after Surgery

- During first post-op visit, remove splint and place in CAM boot.
- Remain NWB on the affected lower extremity.

- Begin AROM/PROM ankle and subtalar joint.
- Begin stretching and strengthening.
- Scar management.
- Continue elevation and ice application.
- Modalities as needed.

6 to 12 weeks after Surgery

- If fracture is clinically and radiographically healed, patient is advanced to WBAT.
- Continue AROM/PROM ankle and subtalar joint.
- Advanced strengthening.
- Modalities as needed.

III. ADMINISTRATIVE TIPS

Although clinical responsibilities in the operating room and outpatient clinic are a large component of Advanced Practice Providers' job, the administrative tasks are just as essential. One may encounter various paperwork including letters of medical necessity, work notes, preauthorizations, FMLA and Workman's compensation forms, along with a variety of time-sensitive disability forms. Completing paperwork and disability forms in an accurate and timely manner increases patient satisfaction and allows for a smooth office workflow.

Tips on Managing the Administrative Workflow

- Create time in your schedule for administrative duties, whether it is a few hours a week or an entire day. During this time, you can concentrate on your administrative work which will improve productivity.
- Create a standardized process for filling out disability forms and handling paperwork to avoid errors and to save time.
- Document telephone calls or any other patient interaction in the medical chart. This enables the rest of the staff to stay updated on patient's current treatment plan and helps "close the loop."

- Create a personalized list of your administrative duties, which may include:
  - Chart completion.
  - Completion of disability forms.
  - Answering patient phone calls or e-mails.
  - Contacting patients with diagnostic test results.
  - Calling patients on post-op day 1 to address any issues or questions.
  - Peer-to-peer phone calls.

IV. WHEN TO DEFER TO THE PHYSICIAN

It is important to know the scope of your practice and understand your limitations. As a health care provider, your goal is to provide optimal care to your patients. Patient care improves with teamwork and effective communication. Staying in close communication with your collaborating physician is essential, especially if you have any patient concerns such as:

- Unclear diagnosis.
- Wound concern (delayed healing, drainage, infection).
- Unexpected finding on physical examination (ie, painful hardware).
- Concerning radiographic finding such as delayed fracture union, nonunion, or hardware failure.
- Anticipated need for surgical intervention.
- When the patient requests to be seen by the physician.

Templating and Documentation

Proper documentation is a crucial component of health care. It ensures continuity of care and serves as a communication tool among providers and staff. Most EMR software are designed with prebuilt templates and default data lists. These templates work best when they are customized to fit the provider's workflow and needs.

Templates that are personalized to the provider's preference improve the ease of documentation, increase charting speed, and quicken the overall workflow. The benefit of adapting the EMR templates to better meet the needs of the practice and the patients may outweigh the additional effort, time, and skill required in creating them.

Tips on Customizing EMR Templates

- Become proficient in your EMR system. Spend time navigating through the available tools and examine how it can fit in your practice workflow.
- Take advantage of the opportunity to sit with EMR project team that may be available to assist you in customizing your personal EMR tools.
- Create preference lists in your EMR to capture common orders such as diagnostic tests, labs, medications, medical supplies, and rehabilitation instructions.
- Spend time adapting the chart note templates to better meet the needs of your practice and patients. Here are some considerations:

  - EMR software are designed with smart links that can pull data such as past medical history, past surgical history, allergies, and current medications from the patient's record into your documentation. Although these tools help make charting patient visit notes easy, fast, and efficient, it is important to verify these data with the patient to avoid errors and capture changes.
  - Create specialty specific templates that capture relevant clinical information. This will help automate the entry of redundant narrative while allowing the provider to key in specific variables about the individual patient.
  - Create personalized "smart-phrases" that can be inserted into your office notes as needed. These may include:
    - Cast application.
    - Injection.

- Suture removal.
- Detailed risks, benefits, and alternatives of surgical procedures.
- Impairment status of patients with worker's compensation insurance.
- Request for prior authorization.

■ Create templates for commonly requested letters and notes. These may include:
  - Letter regarding patient's work status.
  - Letter regarding patient's school attendance and participation in physical education.
  - Excuse letter from jury duty.
  - Letter regarding need for prophylactic antibiotic prior to dental work.
  - Letter of medical necessity for your practice-specific needs (continued physical therapy, dynamic splint, home care, transportation, etc.).

Anticipating Patient's Questions

There are several frequently asked questions from the orthopaedic patient. Anticipating a patient's needs and addressing their questions and concerns is an important component of patient care. The answers to these frequently asked questions may differ based on type of injury, comorbidities, patient's needs, and physician's preference. It is important to have a general idea about how long it takes to recuperate from specific orthopaedic injuries. One must learn the usual duration of incapacity for common orthopaedic conditions seen in the physician's practice. The answers to these commonly asked questions can vary from physician to physician based on their clinical experience and opinion. Thus, it is vital to have a discussion with your collaborating physician when answering these questions. Furthermore, there are additional factors that must be considered in order to answer the patient's questions accurately. Some common questions and potential considerations may include the following:

- "When can I return to work?"
  - Consider patient's job duties.
  - Availability of light duty.
  - Mode of transportation to and from work. (Will the patient be able to manage subway stairs?)
- "How long is the recovery?"
  - The definition of "recovery" varies from patient to patient. For some, it means the ability to return to work. For others, it means return to full function. Ask the patient to define "recovery."
- "When can I drive?" (see Chapter 7 for more information).
  - Discuss with your collaborating physician.
  - Not advised to drive if taking narcotic pain medications.
  - In general, there is no specific guideline. Patients may begin driving when they feel comfortable, safe, and pain free.
- "Do I need general anesthesia?"
  - The choice of anesthesia generally depends on the type of procedure being performed. The choices usually include general anesthesia, regional anesthesia, or local anesthesia with IV sedation. Discuss with your collaborating physician.
  - The ultimate decision for type of anesthesia used is made by the anesthesiologist, who will factor in patient's age, comorbidities, labs, and ECG.
- "How long is the surgery?"
  - Know the common procedures performed in your practice and duration of surgery.
- "When can I shower?"
  - For most arthroscopic procedures, bandages may be removed after 2 to 4 days and the patient is allowed to shower if there are no wound complications. Discuss specific instructions with your collaborating physician.
  - If patient is in a short leg or short arm splint, patient must use a cast cover in the shower to ensure the splint does not get wet.

- "When can I return to sports?"
  - Answer varies widely among physicians and is based on severity of injury, procedure, concomitant injuries, level of participation, and type of sport (contact vs. noncontact).
- "Will I set off metal detectors at the airport?"
  - Depends on location on hardware (deep or superficial) and sensitivity of detectors.
  - Joint replacement patients are no longer given cards identifying the implant. A card or medical documentation no longer exempts a passenger from additional screening.
  - Patients may choose to be screened through imaging technology available at most major airports.
  - If a pat-down is selected, advise the patient to wear clothes that easily allow the patient to reveal surgical scar.

REFERENCES

1. Kramer JF, Dubowitz T, Fowler P, Schachter C, Birmingham T. Functional knee braces and dynamic performance: a review. *Clin J Sports Med*. 1997;7:32-39.
2. Wojtys EM, Kothari SU, Huston LJ. Anterior cruciate ligament functional brace use in sports. *Am J Sports Med*. 1996;24:539-546.
3. Burger RR. Knee braces In: Baker CL, Flandry F, Henderson JM, eds. *The Hughston Clinic Sports Medicine Book*. Baltimore, MD: Williams & Wilkins; 1995:551-558.
4. Liu SH, Mirzayan R. Current review. Functional knee bracing. *Clin Orthop*. 1995;317:273-281.
5. Ott JW, Clancy WG Jr. Functional knee braces. *Orthopedics*. 1993;16:171-175.
6. Beynnon BD, Pope MH, Wertheimer CM, et al. The effect of functional knee-braces on strain on the anterior cruciate ligament in vivo. *J Bone Joint Surg Am*. 1992;74:1298-1312.
7. Maurer SS, Carlin G, Butters R, Scuderi GR. Rehabilitation of the patellofemoral joint. In: ScuderiGR, ed. *The Patella*. New York, NY: Springer-Verlag, 1995:156-159.
8. Shellock FG, Mink JH, Deutsch AL, Molnar T. Effect of a newly designed patellar realignment brace on patellofemoral relationships. *Med Sci Sports Exerc*. 1995;27:469-472.

9. Cutbill JW, Ladly KO, Bray RC, Thorne P, Verhoef M. Anterior knee pain: a review. *Clin J Sports Med*. 1997;7:40-45.
10. Timm KE. Randomized controlled trial of protonics on patellar pain, position, and function. *Med Sci Sports Exerc*. 1998;30:665-70.
11. Arroll B, Ellis-Pegler E, Edwards A, Sutcliffe G. Patellofemoral pain syndrome: a critical review of the clinical trials on nonoperative therapy. *Am J Sports Med*. 1997;25:207-212.
12. Maenpaa H, Lehto MU. Patellar dislocation: the long-term results of nonoperative management in 100 patients. *Am J Sports Med*. 1997;25:213-217.
13. Draganich L, Reider B, Rimington T, Piotrowski G, Mallik K, Nasson S. The effectiveness of self-adjustable custom and off-the-shelf bracing in the treatment of varus gonarthrosis. *J Bone Joint Surg Am*. 2006;88:2645-2652.
14. Self BP, Greenwald RM, Pfaster DS. A biomechanical analysis of a medial unloading brace for osteoarthritis in the knee. *Arthritis Care Res*. 2000;13:191-197.
15. Cerejo R, Dunlop DD, Cahue S, Channin D, Song J, Sharma L. The influence of alignment on risk of knee osteoarthritis progression according to baseline stage of disease. *Arthritis Rheum*. 2002;46:2632-2636.
16. Pollo FE, Jackson RW. Knee bracing for unicompartmental osteoarthritis. *J Am Acad Orthop Surg*. 2006;14:5-11.
17. Squyer E, Stamper DL, Hamilton DT, Sabin JA, Leopold SS. Unloader knee braces for osteoarthritis: do patients actually wear them? *Clin Orthop Relat Res*. 2013; 471(6):1982-1981.
18. Gerber LH. Exercise and arthritis. *Bull Rheum Dis*. 1991;39:1-9
19. McCarthy MR, O'Donoghue PC, Yates CK, Yates-McCarthy JL. The clinical use of continuous passive motion in physical therapy. *J Sport Phys Ther*. 1992;15:132-140.
20. Maniar RN, Baviskar JV, Singhi T, Rathi SS. To use or not use continuous passive motion post total knee or the plastic presenting functional assessment results in early recovery. *J Arthroplasty*. 2012;27(2):193-200.
21. Kerkhoffs GM, Rowe BH, Assendelft WJ, Kelly K, Struijs PA, van Dijk CN. Immobilisation and functional treatment for acute lateral ankle ligament injuries in adults. *Cochrane Database Syst Rev*. 2002;(3):CD003762.
22. Cordova ML, Ingersoll CD, Palmieri RM. Efficacy of prophylactic ankle support: an experimental perspective. *J Athl Train*. 2002;37:446-457.
23. Robbins S, Waked E. Factors associated with ankle injuries. Preventive measures. *Sports Med*. 1998;25(1):63-72.

24. Alvarez RG, Marini A, Schmitt C, Saltzman CL. Stage I and II posterior tibial tendon dysfunction treated by a structured non-operative management protocol: an orthosis and exercise program. *Foot Ankle Int.* 2006;27(1):2-8.

25. Nielsen MD, Dodson EE, Shadrick DL, Catanzariti AR, Mendicino RW, Malay DS. Nonoperative care for the treatment of adult-acquired flatfoot deformity. *J Foot Ankle Surg.* 2011;50(3):311-314.

26. Krause F, Bosshard A, Lehmann O, Weber M. Shell brace for stage II posterior tibial tendon insufficiency. *Foot Ankle Int.* 2008;29(11):1095-1100.

27. Lin JL, Balbas J, Richardson EG. Results of non-surgical treatment of stage II posterior tibial tendon dysfunction: a 7- to 10-year followup. *Foot Ankle Int.* 2008;29(8):781-786.

28. Manufacturing Guidelines. Ankle-foot orthosis. IRSC. 2007. http://www.icrc.org/eng/resources/documents/publication/p0868.htm. Accessed June 15, 2017.

29. Van der Meijden OA, Westgard P, Chandler Z, Gaskill TR, Kokmeyer D, Millett PJ. Rehabilitation after arthroscopic rotator cuff repair: Current concepts review and evidence-based guidelines. *Int J Sports Phys Ther.* 2012;7:197-218.

30. Galkowski V, Brad P, Brian D, David D. Bone stimulation for fracture healing: what's all the fuss? *Indian J Orthop.* 2009;43(2):117-120.

31. Dhurat R, Sukesh MS. Principles and methods of preparation of platelet rich plasma: a review and authors perspective. *J Cutsn Aesthet Surg.* 2014;7(4):189-197.

32. Dockery ML, Wright TW, LaStayo PC. Electromyography of the shoulder: an analysis of passive modes of exercise. *Orthopedics.* 1998;21(11):1181-1184.

33. Smith J, Dahm DL, Kaufman KR, et al. Electromyographic activity in the immobilized shoulder girdle musculature during scapulothoracic exercises. *Arch Phys Med Rehabil.* 2006;87(7):923-927.

34. Adams D, Logerstedt DS, Hunter-Giordano A, Axe MJ, Snyder-Mackler L. Current concepts for anterior cruciate ligament reconstruction: a criterion-based rehabilitation progression. *J Orthop Sports Phys Ther.* 2012;42(7):601-614.

OFFICE PROCEDURES

Kenneth A. Egol

I. INJECTION

An injection may be indicated for either diagnostic or therapeutic purposes such as: rheumatoid arthritis in medium or large joints, osteoarthritis in large weight-bearing joints or the first carpometacarpal joint, other inflammatory arthritis, rotator cuff tendonitis or subdeltoid bursitis, trochanteric bursitis, carpal tunnel syndrome, De Quervain's tendonitis, trigger finger, lateral epicondylitis, trigger point pain, etc.[1]

Common injectable agents:

- Steroids[2,3]:
  - Glucocorticoids: Methylprednisolone
    - Large joints (knee, ankle, shoulder): 20 to 80 mg
    - Medium joints (elbow, wrist): 10 to 40 mg
    - Small joints (MCP, IP, SC, AC joints): 4 to 10 mg
  - Corticosteroids: Triamcinolone acetonide (maximum dose/treatment including polyarticular injection 80 mg) 40 mg = 1 mL
    - Larger joints: 5 to 15 mg for the initial injection and up to 40 mg for subsequent injections
    - Smaller joints: 2.5 to 5 mg for the initial injection and up to 10 mg for subsequent injections
- Local anesthetics:
  - Lidocaine: Onset of action: 1 to 2 minutes, duration: 1 hour, dose: maximum 4.5 mg/kg/dose not to exceed 300 mg; do not repeat within 2 hours, usually between 3 and 8 mL for

large–medium joint injections, 0.5 mL for tendon sheath injections

■ Bupivacaine: Onset of action: 30 minutes, duration: 8 hours

Frequency of Injection

It is recommended to limit intra-articular glucocorticoid injections overall; however, safe rates of injection range from four lifetime injections per joint for osteoarthritis (no sooner than every 3 months) to one injection per month per joint (not to exceed four injections in a year) with severe rheumatoid arthritis.[4]

Potential Complications

Cellulitis, septic joint, and local muscle inflammation. There is controversial evidence regarding the systemic effect of intra-articular glucocorticoids on bone metabolism, patients on therapeutic anticoagulation, tendon rupture (decreased when glucocorticoid is mixed with local anesthetic), nerve atrophy/necrosis, skin atrophy, hypopigmentation (especially in patients with darker pigmentation).

Procedure

Gloves are required. As this is a sterile procedure, a sterile field is required. Examine and palpate the site, then mark the site of injection with marker or by making an impression. Next prepare the skin with several concentric outward spirals of either a chlorhexidine or an iodine prep. Once the skin is prepped, do not touch the site of injection again with unsterile finger as skin will need to be prepared again. Next apply local anesthetic if indicated. Ethyl chloride spray or a subcutaneous wheel of lidocaine (use a 22-gauge needle) may be administered to reduce injection site pain. Anesthetic may also be mixed with the glucocorticoid injection. For intra-articular injections, drawback on your syringe before injection to confirm you are not intravascular. Administer the medication, remove the needle following sharps safety guidelines, and apply gentle pressure to site with gauze. Apply a Band-Aid or dressing over the site of injection.

Patient Education

Advise patients to decrease weight bearing and strenuous activities for 48 hours. Patients may apply ice to the injected joint and should be instructed to observe the area for any significant rebound swelling, erythema, warmth, fever, worsening pain, and drainage from the injection site. Ice may be beneficial in the period between inactivity of local anesthetic and onset of steroid action.[1]

II. ASPIRATION (ARTHROCENTESIS)

Indications

An aspiration, or arthrocentesis, may be indicated for either diagnostic or therapeutic purposes. Arthrocentesis and/or analysis of synovial fluid (to rule out a septic joint or diagnose gout), to relieve pressure, and cyst aspiration (ganglion, Baker's).

Needle Size

An 18- to 20-gauge needle is recommended for most large joint aspirations. For smaller joints, such as the wrist or IP joints, a smaller needle, such as a 22- to 24-gauge needle, is recommended.

Syringe Size

For obviously large joint effusions, a 20 mL syringe is recommended, otherwise a 10 to 12 mL syringe should be adequate for shoulder and knee aspirations, or a 5 mL syringe for smaller joints or ganglion cysts. Have additional syringes available in the situation where your syringe fills.

III. COMMON APPROACHES TO INJECTION OR ARTHROCENTESIS

The key to all procedures is to avoid bone and neurovascular bundles. Mark and prepare the site as described earlier. Following injection or aspiration, apply gentle pressure to site and affix a dressing in place.

Posterior Glenohumeral Approach

Externally rotate the shoulder. Mark two finger breadths distal to the scapular spine and two finger breadths medial to the acromial edge. In this "soft spot" direct the needle anteriorly and medially until you puncture the posterior shoulder capsule (Figure 11-1).

Subacromial Approach

Palpate and mark the posterolateral corner of the acromion process. Next palpate the edge of the bone and mark as the injection site. Direct the needle perpendicular to the skin through the deltoid muscle just under the acromion aiming toward the AC joint (Figure 11-2).

Lateral Elbow

Flex the elbow to 90 degrees. Draw a triangle from the radial head, lateral epicondyle, and tip of the olecranon. Direct the needle perpendicular to the skin into the center of the triangle about 2 to 2.5 cm deep (Figure 11-3).

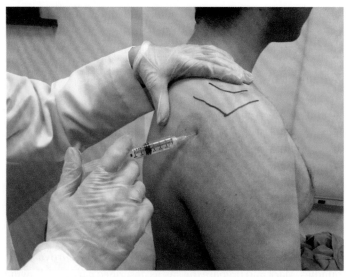

Figure 11-1 Posterior glenohumeral injection. Shoulder marking delineates scapular spine and acromion anatomic position.

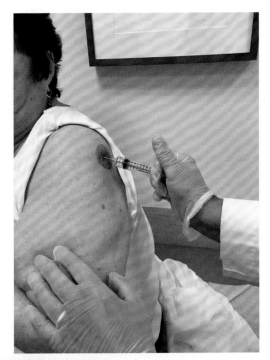

Figure 11-2 **Subacromial injection.** Shoulder marking delineates posterolateral acromial anatomic positon.

Dorsal Approach to Wrist

Instruct the patient to flex their wrist. Palpate Lister's tubercle. Mark the point just distal to this and ulnar to the anatomic snuffbox (between the third and fourth extensor compartments). Insert the needle perpendicular to the skin (Figure 11-4).

Superolateral Knee Approach

Instruct the patient to lie supine with their knee extended. Flex the knee about 15 degrees and support with a bump. Direct the needle toward the center of the patella, then slightly posteriorly and inferomedially into the knee joint (Figure 11-5).

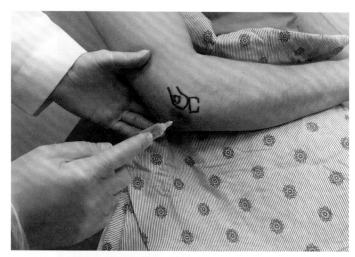

Figure 11-3 Elbow injection (lateral). Elbow marking delineates lateral epicondyle capitulum and radial head anatomic position.

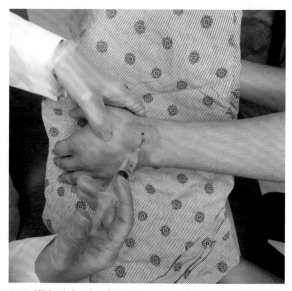

Figure 11-4 Wrist injection (dorsal approach). Blue dot points to the anatomic position of the dorsal radius tubercle, or Lister's tubercle.

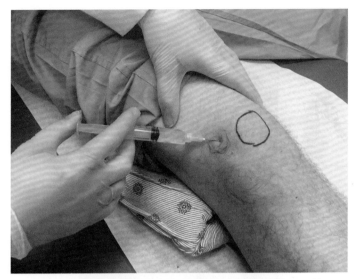

Figure 11-5 Superolateral intra-articular knee injection. Knee marking delineates the patella. The injection site is at the lateral aspect of the suprapatellar pouch.

Anteromedial Knee Approach

Instruct the patient with their lower leg hung over the edge of the examination table with their knee flexed 90 degrees. Mark medial to the patella tendon and at the joint line. Direct the needle perpendicular to the skin, parallel to the plateau, and about 45 degrees toward the midline (Figure 11-6).

Ankle Approach

With the foot in dorsiflexion, mark just medial to the anterior tibialis tendon and just lateral to medial malleolus. Direct the needle posteriorly (Figure 11-7).

IV. LABORATORY EVALUATION

A standard workup to rule out a septic joint includes sending synovial fluid aspirate for aerobic/anaerobic and fungal culture and

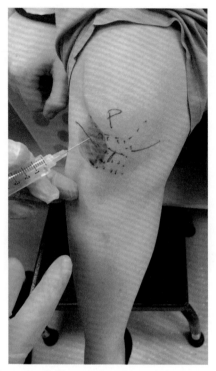

Figure 11-6 **Anteromedial intra-articular knee injection.** Knee marking "P" delineates patella, "T" delineates patellar tendon, and the solid lines delineate joint line.

sensitivity, white blood cell count, and crystal examination under polarized light. Note the gross appearance of the fluid, the volume of fluid aspirated, as well as the patients' pre- and postprocedure pain scores. Additional tips:

V. TIPS AND TRICKS

- Ultrasonography may be used to guide intra-articular shoulder and knee injections. A referral to an interventional radiologist

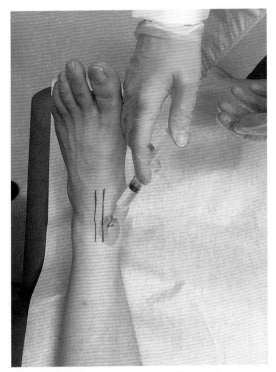

Figure 11-7 Ankle injection. Ankle marking delineates the anatomic position of the tibialis anterior tendon.

is recommended for intra-articular hip and sacroiliac joint injections. Single-use medication vials are preferred to multidose vials to prevent contamination.

- In the event of a dry tap with high suspicion for a septic joint, attempt the aspiration from another anatomic approach.
- It is generally safe to perform arthorocentesis on patients therapeutically anticoagulated. It is recommended that smaller gauge needles are utilized.
- It is not recommended to shave hair at the procedure site owing to increased exposure of staphylococci. If there is a high hair burden, scissors may be used to trim the site.

VI. SUTURE/STAPLE REMOVAL

Timing of suture or staple removal will vary based on the anatomic site and the presence of comorbidities (diabetes, peripheral vascular disease)/therapies (systemic steroids, chemotherapy, DMARDs) affecting patients' ability to heal. Most upper and lower extremity incisions are well healed and may have sutures/staples removed on postoperative days 7 through 14. Incisions over extensor surfaces and areas of high tension may be left in place closer to 14 days. Educate your patient that this procedure is relatively painless. They may feel a tugging sensation as a suture is removed or a pinch as a staple is removed. Empower the patient by letting them know if at any time they need a break from suture/staple removal to let you know. First apply nonsterile gloves then assess the wound for healing and adequate skin approximation. Some wounds may be healing well but may need additional time to prevent dehiscence. In this situation, every other or every third suture/staple may be removed. After assessing the condition of the wound, prepare the skin with a chlorhexidine or betadine solution. Then use sterile forceps to grasp either the knot or tail of the suture while gently lifting away from the skin surface (Figure 11-8). Sterile suture scissors or a #11 blade scalpel may be used to cut the suture. Remove the loosened suture with the forceps. For staples, a sterile staple remover should be utilized. Place the tips of the device around the staple, then apply pressure to close the handles together (Figure 11-9). The staple will straighten, allowing you to lift the staple from the skin. Have a sterile 4 × 4 nearby as suture/staple holes may ooze blood. Once all sutures/staples are removed, you may again cleanse the wound. Then apply an adhesive solution such as Benzoin or Mastisol around the incision. Once the adhesive dries you may apply adhesive strips with tension to bring wound edges together to provide additional strength to the healing wound. If at any point during the procedure the wound edges gap/open, discontinue the removal procedure and apply adhesive strips. Educate the patient on wound care instructions as well as when they may shower. Incisions should not be scrubbed but rather cleansed gently. It